HIV Pioneers

HIV PIONEERS

LIVES LOST, CAREERS CHANGED, *and* SURVIVAL

Edited by WENDEE M. WECHSBERG
Foreword by James W. Curran

JOHNS HOPKINS UNIVERSITY PRESS

Baltimore

RTI Press / RTI International
Research Triangle Park, North Carolina

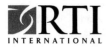

RTI Press publication No. BK-0021-1801
https://doi.org/10.3768/rtipress.2018.bk.0021.1801
www.rti.org/rtipress

The RTI Press mission is to disseminate information about RTI research, analytic tools, and technical expertise to a national and international audience. RTI Press publications are peer-reviewed by at least two independent substantive experts and one or more Press editors.
    RTI International is an independent, nonprofit research organization dedicated to improving the human condition. We combine scientific rigor and technical expertise in social and laboratory sciences, engineering, and international development to deliver solutions to the critical needs of clients worldwide.

This publication is part of the RTI Press Book series.
RTI International
3040 East Cornwallis Road, PO Box 12194
Research Triangle Park, NC 27709-2194, USA
rtipress@rti.org   www.rti.org

To the lives lost and to the unborn babies and

young women we hope to protect

CONTENTS

FOREWORD

Where were you in 1981? When did you first learn of AIDS? For many of us involved in public health, healthcare, or research, the answer to those questions marks a personal and professional turning point. This book captures the life-changing experiences from dozens of those who were and remain deeply committed to battling the global HIV pandemic. Wendee M. Wechsberg has been there from the start, and here she has expertly captured the varied, compelling, and historically significant stories of many HIV pioneers.

On June 5, 1981, five cases of *Pneumocystis carinii* pneumonia were reported in previously healthy homosexual men from Los Angeles, California. These cases represented the first published reports of what became the global HIV/AIDS pandemic. During the next few years, discoveries were rapid. The epidemiologic patterns were clearly delineated, leading to consensus recommendations for prevention in 1982 and 1983, even before the cause of AIDS was found. In 1983–1984, the AIDS virus was isolated and proved to be causal. Defying predictions, in 1986–1987 the first antiretroviral drug, AZT, was shown to be at least partially effective. Isolation of HIV and the availability of diagnostic tests allowed better determination of the natural history of the disease and of the global extent of the epidemic. Progress has continued in the following decades, especially with the discovery of HAART (highly active antiretroviral therapy), further advances in diagnostics, and the effectiveness of antiretroviral (ARV) therapy for prevention and care. Activism by community members and providers alike, including many of these authors, has been crucial to establishing priorities and guiding progress. Importantly, effective ARV therapy has been provided to over 18 million persons worldwide.

But biologic and social factors continue to threaten progress and favor long-term endemicity. The virus itself persists for the life of the host and has eluded efforts to develop a curative therapy or a vaccine. Discrimination based on homophobia, racism, sexism, poverty, and the infection itself is a constant factor to be faced in every community.

The Joint United Nations Programme on HIV/AIDS (UNAIDS) estimates that 35 million persons have lost their lives to HIV, and of the 37 million people now living with HIV, fewer than half are diagnosed and in care. More than 2 million people became newly infected in 2015.

Much has been accomplished in the first 35 years, but much work remains to be done by science and society. HIV pioneers are more than survivors; they are also committed veterans engaged for the future. We can take inspiration from them and from the late Dr. Jonathan Mann, our esteemed colleague, who was a global leader in the AIDS battle from 1984 until 1998. He founded Project SIDA in Zaire in 1984 and started the World Health Organization Global Programme on AIDS in 1986. From there he persistently linked the fight against HIV to the pursuit of human rights. Shortly before he and his wife perished in an airplane crash in 1998, he had addressed the 12th International Conference on AIDS in Geneva. He said:

> Our responsibility is historic. For when the history of AIDS and the global response is written, our most precious contribution may well be that, at a time of plague, we did not flee, we did not hide, we did not separate ourselves.

Read these personal narratives. They will touch you deeply and hopefully inspire you to continue or to join the ongoing fight against HIV in your community and in the world.

James W. Curran
Dean of Public Health
Professor of Epidemiology
Co-Director, Emory Center for AIDS Research
Emory University
Atlanta, Georgia

INTRODUCTION

WENDEE M. WECHSBERG

WE KNOW THAT TREMENDOUS STRIDES have been made in the prevention and treatment of HIV since the epidemic first appeared in the early 1980s with the discovery of HIV. Today there is considerable scientific and public dialogue about the possible end of the AIDS epidemic. However, it is important not to forget where we've come from. Since HIV was first identified, many of the early public health pioneers are gone and some of the early stories from the field are at risk of being lost, including survivor stories.

I was at an AIDS meeting two years ago when I heard one of the pioneers from India, Suniti Solomon, had passed. It was because of her sad passing that I thought to put together this book. Her son did a tribute to her at the AIDS 2016 conference in Durban, South Africa, but found it was too painful to write her story for this volume. Personally, I can say she was the true pioneer in India and was gracious to me when I had a sabbatical there almost a decade ago. I witnessed firsthand Dr. Solomon's impact in her clinics serving the most vulnerable people.

Also, some years earlier, we lost James A. Inciardi, a very prominent figure in the addiction field and a good friend. Jim contributed many seminal books and articles, especially about crack cocaine, criminal justice, and sex workers. I remember him with fond memories from our many meetings as part of the National Institute on Drug Abuse's Cooperative Agreement for HIV AIDS risk-reduction studies in the mid-1990s. We were committed to issues on gender and worked together starting new projects for women, even though, as I often rebuked him good naturedly, he was the traditional Italian male. Most importantly, he had the heart and the head for the work to be impactful.

HIV Pioneers is a collection of national and global "first stories" from the outset of the AIDS epidemic and the discovery of HIV. Contributors include prominent HIV scientists, leaders, and survivors who provide a broad range of historical perspectives, including the impact that the epidemic had on our careers, how governments responded, how research agendas were developed, and how AIDS service agencies started and case management was developed. These narratives capture the multiple voices and experiences of those still working diligently and innovatively in the field, voices from survivors, and those of historical figures who have passed the public health baton to others to carry on the fight against HIV. Many of these people are also activists and concerned for the well-being of their patients, family, and friends. Because of my own personal story and my professional start in clinical addiction treatment in 1977, many of the authors are people I have known all these years in the field, and I am grateful they agreed to be part of this book.

It is important to note that this collection of stories is not the total picture. Many people I asked to contribute found that they were unable to share their reflections at this time. However, I attempted to present stories from across the United States and some important ones globally from those who were there from the beginning. Some may be controversial, but I tried to make sure these stories were told, especially from the early days so they are not forgotten. Also, the survivors' stories often teach us the most poignant lessons about humanity and womanity, as some still face bias and struggle every day, so their courage continues to be profound.

Some of these narratives are very personal, some reflect initial research developments, and some are critical historical government accounts not only shedding light on the experiences of these pioneers but also preserving valuable lessons learned that can potentially be applied to future epidemics.

My most sincere thank-you goes to Jeffrey Novey, my editor at RTI, who worked diligently with me throughout this project when so much seemed to be on our plate that we might never be done.

But Not All
More than thirty years ago,
fear, panic, isolation, stigma, and death.
So many lives.
Time provides wisdom, knowledge, and tools.
We are getting it.
But not all.

HIV now a chronic condition in high-income countries.
Not so elsewhere.
Women in low- and middle-income countries getting HIV more than men;
gender roles, rape, and little choice in vocation.
But not all.
Testing more, better medication, pushing adherence.
But not all.
Still fighting fear, stigma, ignorance, and poverty.
Food security comes first;
families still go to bed hungry.
Implementing programs to empower, to link, to case manage, to track, to
    support.
But not all.
Deeply rooted societal gender inequality and cultural roles.
Keeping women vulnerable and voiceless against brutality and sexual
    control.
But not all.
Reaching through implementers, working for sustainability.
But never for all.
More than thirty years on, untold miles traveled, learning, helping, training,
    implementing, mentoring.
Many deaths, many very personal.
Poignant stories of survival and lessons learned keep us going.
Promoting life, equality, and access to healthcare.
Being healthy, staying HIV free.
But not all, never all.
We have not reached them all.
We are not done.

—WENDEE M. WECHSBERG

Patients, Physicians, and Hospitals

The Healer, Dr. Beny Primm

Uncommon Man for Uncommon Times

WARREN W. HEWITT JR.

C.S. LEWIS, the noted English writer and poet, once said, "Extraordinary things only happen to extraordinary people. Maybe it's a sign that you've got an extraordinary destiny—something greater than you could've imagined." In Harlem, there was such a man who worked on being extraordinary throughout his life and as a result was responsible for extraordinary accomplishments that changed the course of two devastating epidemics.

In 1963, a young Black physician, Dr. Beny J. Primm, began his first full-time medical position as an anesthesiologist at Harlem Hospital. Looking forward to a life's career as a hospital anesthesiologist, he discovered that most of the people he saw in the operating room who had acute puncture wound trauma were also drug users. He realized that the task of medical care could not be fully completed on the surgical table because the nexus for these traumatic injuries was in reality a constellation of social and health-care problems that had a disproportionate impact on the health and well-being of many Harlem residents. This sobering reality dramatized the gravity of the drug abuse problem and the need for effective care in Harlem.

The reality of these issues ultimately led Dr. Primm to rethink his long-term medical goals and to make a professional and life changing commitment to find the means to arrest the devastation that the drug abuse epidemic was having in Harlem. Unknown to him at the time, the magnitude of this apocalyptical devastation was only a precursor for what was yet to come.

The Landscape of AIDS

The landscape for the AIDS epidemic among injecting drug users and for the people of Harlem was established long before AIDS was formally recognized as a public health issue. In 1964, Harlem had the dubious distinction of being the drug capital of America, with drug abuse rates nearly 10 times higher than the whole of New York City and 12 times higher than the total United States. At this time, only a few drug abuse treatment programs existed in New York and there were virtually none in the primarily Black and Hispanic communities of Harlem and Bedford Stuyvesant in Brooklyn. The persona of the addict became not only a public anathema, but it was also a convenient focal point for political diatribes to ramp up public support for more law enforcement solutions to the so-called war on drugs. For addicts in New York, this hostile political climate forced them to "go to ground" and to find unseen alleys and off-the-beaten-track buildings to shoot up. This unsympathetic climate toward addicts would later become a serious impediment during the AIDS epidemic when efforts were made to provide AIDS services and outreach to injection drug users in Harlem and throughout New York City.

At Harlem Hospital, Dr. Primm was appointed to head the Narcotics Control Program, but he quickly realized that to meet the needs of the addicts in Harlem he would need to secure community support as well as support from the addicts of Harlem. At this point in his medical career, he had to buttress his medical training with a new set of skills that would allow him to lead, organize, advocate, and sometimes agitate on behalf of the addicts of Harlem. From his daunting challenges with how to provide effective treatment in Harlem emerged a philosophy of drug treatment that would become his raison d'être and his life's work—and the basis for how he would ultimately approach the coming intersection of an old and new epidemic in Harlem and in Brooklyn.

After extensive research and consultation with Drs. Jerry Jaffee, Herb Kleber, and Ed Senay, as well as a host of researchers and clinicians, on the question of how best to treat the heroin addict, Dr. Primm found himself faced with the necessity to rethink his earlier objections to long-term methadone maintenance. He found that methadone maintenance allowed many addicts to transform their lives, have families, become gainfully employed, and not return to heroin use. More importantly, he subsequently realized that he had discovered a vehicle for drug abuse treatment that would pay enormous dividends in the upcoming AIDS epidemic among the residents of Harlem and Brooklyn.

In 1969, Dr. Primm founded the Addiction Research and Treatment Center (ARTC), the first Black-managed methadone maintenance treatment program, which would subsequently become the largest minority-operated not-for-profit drug treatment program in the United States.[1] Though ARTC was

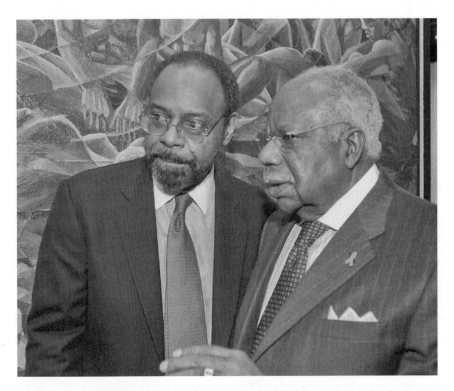

FIGURE 1.1. Dr. Beny Primm (*right*) with Mr. Richard Jones, Executive Dean for Accreditation & Quality Assurance at Medgar Evers College, CUNY. Photo taken at the Addiction Research and Treatment Corp (ARTC) in Brooklyn, NY. Photo courtesy of the Primm family.

to be a beacon of hope to addicts in Harlem and Brooklyn and throughout the New York boroughs, it was also a target for many detractors who believed that methadone was merely substitution of one addicting drug for another—or worse, who saw methadone maintenance in conspiratorial terms, a directed threat to the Black community. Mostly, the opposition came from those who were most opposed to drug treatment being located in their communities—NIMBYs (or "not in my backyard"). Ironically, many of those who stood to benefit from treatment were from families in these communities who were among the most opposed to locating treatment in their communities. ARTC, from inception, was a grand experiment in community-based treatment for addicts; but as history would write, it became so much more than merely a drug treatment program. It became a model not only for drug abuse treatment but also for comprehensive, integrated care.

The dawn of the AIDS epidemic occurred a little less than six months after Ronald Reagan was sworn in as the 40th president of the United States. The first reported cases of *Pneumocystis carinii* pneumonia (*P. carinii*) reported among gay men[2] and drug abusers[3] had no significance for the new administration. While the epidemic had not been recognized as a matter of national public concern, it could not have come at a worse moment in time.

The incoming administration's populist-grounded philosophy, characterized as "New Federalism," adopted the view that funding decisions were better made by state and local governments than the federal government. The administration opposed what they termed "Big Government," meaning a big federal government. Consequently, for the drug abuse field, this translated into the consolidation and reduction of all drug, alcohol, and mental health categorical funds into a single Block Grant.[4,5] These changes in federal policy in decision-making for drug abuse from federal to state and local governments would become an important impediment to future efforts made to develop a coherent, integrated strategy to address the intersecting epidemics of drug abuse and AIDS.

By the early 1980s, a profound trend had become apparent among the injecting drug users in Harlem and Brooklyn. Mortality had been rising at alarming rates, heretofore unheard of among injecting drug users and not likely a result of overdoses based on the changes in the purity of street heroin. AIDS had come to Harlem. By 1984–1985, nearly 40 percent of ARTC's patients were positive with HTLV-III (the earlier designation of the virus causing AIDS).[1] The alarm created throughout New York City, and especially among drug treatment programs, rose to near panic levels.

In response to this growing concern in the treatment field, Dr. Primm, now the director of ARTC, brought together the New York drug treatment community as well as a number of physicians and local politicians to consider how best to respond. Though the public seemed convinced that AIDS was a "gay disease," Dr. Primm knew otherwise. Based on what he was seeing in his own program, throughout the city, and around the country, he knew that HIV/AIDS was directly connected to drug abusers and specifically to those who injected heroin and shared their "works" with other heroin users. However, he harbored visceral fear that the number of individuals infected would increasingly come from the Black populations of Harlem and Brooklyn. His fears were not unfounded.

A New Vision for Treatment

By orchestrating efforts to prevent HIV/AIDS among drug users by getting them stabilized on methadone maintenance, Dr. Primm realized that ARTC could continue to have a modest impact on the HIV/AIDS epidemic. However, in light of these disturbing trends throughout New York City, he recognized that the enormity of this epidemic would necessitate the creation of new, locally based collaborations with a variety of people and organizations. So in 1986, he created the Brooklyn AIDS Task Force to be that collective community effort to address all aspects of HIV/AIDS in the Borough of Brooklyn. It also marked his personal transformation from a physician treating addicts to a physician treating a community. As an advocate, organizer, and a leader he offered guidance and vision in an effort to arrest the dual specters of substance abuse and HIV/AIDS in the Black and Hispanic communities of New York City.

By early 1987, it had become apparent to Dr. Primm that issues being addressed at the national level often overlooked the interests/needs of Blacks and other minorities. He realized that a national voice was needed to articulate the agenda and strategic direction specifically relevant to the needs of minority communities. In 1987, he was one of several people who were instrumental in founding the National Minority AIDS Council (NMAC), which would ultimately become the national voice for action related to minority people.

Later that year, on June 29, 1987, President Reagan signed Executive Order 12601, establishing the Commission on the Human Immunodeficiency Virus Epidemic.[6] As a preeminent expert on substance abuse treatment and as a medical doctor familiar with AIDS in the highly affected areas in New York City, Dr. Primm was invited by the president to become a member of the Commission on HIV. As the sole Black member of the commission with tangible experience and understanding of substance abuse/addiction treatment, he was instrumental in informing and guiding the deliberations of the commission on the treatment of addiction. The commission's final report reflected a number of key themes Dr. Primm had advocated for during the closed deliberations by the commission members and also a recommendation made as part of the Coolfont Conference (a US Public Health Service meeting of AIDS experts at the Coolfont Conference Center in West Virginia in 1986).[7] The commission urged the president to provide funding to support a major expansion of drug treatment programs. More importantly, the commission acknowledged that to reduce the spread of HIV among injecting drug users, a simple expansion of drug treatment capacity alone would not suffice.

Consequently, they also recommended that national drug abuse policy incorporate "treatment on demand" as a basic tenet of drug treatment programs.[8]

Crack Changes the Landscape

When "crack cocaine" came to Harlem in the mid-1980s, the landscape of drug abuse changed in a dramatic fashion. ARTC, like many drug treatment programs in New York City, was in a quandary about how to approach treatment for the increasing population of crack cocaine–addicted drug users. Conventional psychiatric and drug abuse treatment models designed to treat heroin addiction were not effective for the crack cocaine addict. Also, many crack users were using other drugs and had co-occurring mental health disorders. Relapse rates were higher than they had ever been. Cheap crack cocaine, which was highly addictive, produced a sudden and intense euphoria, extreme craving, and compulsive drug-seeking behavior. Crack was not just another drug, but a street commodity widely sold in Black and Hispanic communities and often punctuated by violent competition.

As crack insinuated itself into Harlem and Brooklyn, Dr. Primm began to see the emergence of a new and disturbing drug abuse pattern. What he observed from his vantage point at ARTC gave him pause and an irrepressible fear that the crack epidemic in New York City and other urban centers would transform the HIV epidemic as the number of crack addicts increased. He realized how great the vulnerability for HIV infection could be in many of these cloistered, even segregated, communities where the widespread practice of trading sex for drugs was increasing at near-exponential levels.[9,10]

This new epidemic of crack use rapidly overtook heroin as the number one drug problem from coast to coast. As the number of new crack users increased, so did the demand for drug treatment. In 1988, presidential candidate George H. W. Bush invited Dr. Primm to discuss his thoughts on how to shape candidate Bush's agenda to address the increasing growth of crack cocaine in communities across the country. He quickly outlined a list of recommendations that had been presented to former President Reagan by his Commission on HIV, including expanding substance abuse treatment programs and implementing "treatment on demand." He also pointed out that retaining crack cocaine abusers in drug treatment could be extremely beneficial as a secondary prevention strategy for HIV. In 1989, after George H. W. Bush became the 41st president of the United States, Dr. Primm was installed in the Department of Health and Human Services to lead the newly established Office for Treatment Improvement in the Substance Abuse and Mental Health Services Administration.

Three years later when he left the Office for Treatment Improvement, he had succeeded in expanding drug abuse treatment programs (consistent with the recommendations of the Reagan Commission on HIV) to address crack cocaine and other drug problems in local communities. He introduced a new standard of comprehensive care for drug abuse treatment programs predicated on the provision of what he characterized as a "supermarket of services" designed to meet the individual addict's need for services. He forged linkages between drug abuse treatment programs and primary care and AIDS service organizations, and incorporated HIV identification and outreach services into the fabric of drug abuse treatment. Finally, with the recognition of the terrible burden of disease that crack cocaine was having on women, especially Black and other minority women, he directed the development of the first generation of gender-focused residential treatment programs for pregnant and postpartum women and their children, as well as programs for other women and their children.[11]

The Minority AIDS Initiative

By 1996, many of the patients in Dr. Primm's program who were HIV positive were also receiving the latest generation of drugs to combat HIV. High rates of mortality that had characterized clients in treatment at ARTC during the early years of the epidemic had dropped substantially during this period. The new non-nucleoside reverse transcriptase inhibitor (NNRTI) drug and combination antiretroviral therapy (ART) drugs had made it possible for those living with HIV to live longer and healthier lives with renewed hope. By 1997, AIDS mortality had slowed substantially, based on more aggressive and early treatment with highly active antiretroviral therapy (HAART).

In March 1998, Dr. Primm was invited to attend a meeting at the Centers for Disease Control and Prevention (CDC) in Atlanta, where the CDC staff presented data showing that the AIDS mortality among African Americans was nearly 10 times greater than among Whites. Based on post-meeting discussions, the attendees prepared a list of demands directed to CDC. As the spokesman for those assembled at the meeting, Dr. Primm prefaced his list of the demands by conveying his outrage, calling the situation a "national public disaster, a national health disaster." He took these demands that had been given to CDC to Washington, DC, and presented them to Representative Nancy Pelosi and Congressional Black Caucus Members Louis Stokes and Maxine Waters, and from there to the Secretary of Health and Human Services, Donna Shalala. Given Dr. Primm's tenacity and commitment, on October 28, 1998, President Clinton announced the Minority HIV/AIDS Initiative, citing that "AIDS is a particularly severe and ongoing crisis in the African-American and Hispanic communities and in other communities of color."[12]

For Dr. Primm, the Minority AIDS Initiative was the culmination of his personal journey grounded in his commitment to address an epidemic that had moved his spirit and heart from his early days in Harlem.

An Extraordinary Destiny

This extraordinary physician, the founder of ARTC, and a man of great compassion and conviction accomplished so much in a rich life of service to the people he cared so much about—the addicts, the disenfranchised, those at risk for and living with HIV, and Black gay men. His ideas inspired fundamental changes in the texture of American policies directed at arresting the AIDS epidemic. My dearest friend, Dr. Beny J. Primm, died October 16, 2015. He is survived by his family and friends, literally thousands of Harlem and Brooklyn addicts whom he helped to overcome their addictions, and countless thousands in this country and abroad who were inspired to act on behalf of others because of the passion of this truly extraordinary man.

References

1. Primm BJ, Friedman JS. The healer: a doctor's crusade against addiction and AIDS. Charleston, SC: CreateSpace Publishing; 2014.

2. Centers for Disease Control. *Pneumocystis* pneumonia—Los Angeles. MMWR Morb Mortal Wkly Rep. 1981;30(21):250–2.

3. Masur H, Michelis MA, Greene JB, Onorato I, Vande Stouwe RA, Holzman RS et al. An outbreak of community-acquired *Pneumocystis carinii* pneumonia: initial manifestation of cellular immune dysfunction. N Engl J Med 1981;305(24):1431–8.

4. Axelrod D. State government: block in health. Bull N Y Acad Med 1983 Jan–Feb;59(1):75–81.

5. Brandt EN, Jr. Block grants and the resurgence of federalism. Public Health Rep 1981 Nov–Dec;96(6):495–7.

6. Exec. Order No. 12601, Presidential Commission on the Human Immunodeficiency Virus Epidemic, 3 C.F.R. (1987), as amended by EO 12603.

7. Public Health Service's Executive Task Force on AIDS. Coolfont report: a PHS plan for prevention and control of AIDS and AIDS virus. Public Health Rep 1986 Jul–Aug;101(4):341–8.

8. Presidential Commission on the Human Immunodeficiency Virus Epidemic. Report of the Presidential Commission on the Human Immunodeficiency Syndrome Virus Epidemic. Washington, DC: The Commission; 1988.

9. Edlin BR, Irwin KL, Faruque S, McCoy CB, Word C, Serrano Y et al.; Multicenter Crack Cocaine and HIV Infection Study Team. Intersecting epidemics—crack cocaine use and HIV infection among inner-city young adults. N Engl J Med 1994;331(21):1422–7. https://doi.org/10.1056/NEJM1994 11243312106

10. Primm BJ. AIDS: today's and tomorrow's crisis. J Health Care Poor Underserved 1990;1(1):185–95 discussion 196–202.

11. Zweben JE, ed. An interview with Beny Primm, MD, Director, Center for Substance Abuse Treatment. J Psychoactive Drugs 1993;25(1):1–4. https://doi.org /10.1080/02791072.1993.10472585

12. Clinton WJ. Remarks announcing the HIV/AIDS initiative in minority communities. Weekly Compilation of Presidential Documents 1998 Oct 28;34(44): 2166–2168.

"That AZT Kills Patients"

Learning from Lamar—A 25-Year-Long Patient-Doctor Relationship

JEFFREY SAMET

1992: "Doc—I have the virus."

2016: "Who would've thought that I would be alive today?"

T O A NEW GENERAL INTERNAL medicine physician faculty member at Boston City Hospital in 1989, opportunities to improve the quality of care for patients who sought medical attention at the public hospital seemed endless. Having trained the past 10 years in Houston (Baylor College of Medicine, Ben Taub Hospital) and then Boston to become a card-carrying physician, two looming medical care challenges seemed unavoidable and fascinating to me, HIV infection and addiction. These diseases confronted one at every turn, working on the hospital wards and in the medical clinics. The presentation of a patient for the first time in the outpatient setting for HIV care in those days was a recipe for disaster. The reality was that our medical care system was poorly equipped to address the needs of an individual coming into care at that moment in time in their life.

Imagine the difficulty of deciding to go to the doctor and saying, "I need help. I tested positive for HIV." Medical care was a strange maze that once entered might never be exited vertically. As one patient said, "I don't want to leave here in a box, Doc."

Imagine being the doctor who often felt alone and inadequate to deal with the other problems that so commonly coexisted with the "diagnosis." Even a 40-minute new patient appointment was thrown into bedlam when the "problem list" for this new patient with HIV infection transformed into a nightmarish array of challenging-to-treat diagnoses.

Lamar was typical in that way. He presented to medical care with challenges greater than his mere HIV infection. Other potentially more important problems were his heroin dependence, injection drug use, depressive symptoms, chronic pain, legal problems, unstable housing, and poor social support. He was also wary of a medical care system that was big, mostly white, confusing, and although fortunately available in Massachusetts, not necessarily aligned with his needs and preferences.

In 1992, Lamar was a 38-year-old African American man who had been addicted to heroin for just about half of his life. Despite that burden, he had gained highly valued skills as a sought-after auto mechanic. He had a steady girlfriend. He had stayed up on the news about the HIV epidemic and sought HIV testing, realizing that his behaviors put him in a high-risk group and understanding that this was an issue worthy of his attention. Consequently, he sought out medical evaluation in our relatively new clinic established at Boston City Hospital to try to meet the needs of the complex HIV-infected patient trying to establish medical care, the HIV Diagnostic Evaluation Unit. Referred to as the DEU, this inconspicuously named weekly clinic took all comers and provided relatively rapid access to medical care (within a week) for anyone with HIV infection. The beauty of the clinic was that it had a team-based structure in an era when team-based care was not part of the medical vernacular. The key team members were the full-time committed nurse, the full-time committed social worker, and the medical directors (with our one-day-a-week commitment), along with medical trainees who rotated through the clinic for one weekly half-day shift, four weeks at a time.

Lamar presented to this 2-year-old clinic back in 1992, seeking help and feeling skeptical. Engagement was the essence of what we did in the DEU. That goal was accomplished after a couple of weeks, typically including two DEU multidisciplinary medical appointments as well as multiple specific nursing and social worker appointments. After a complete medical evaluation, including HIV clinical and laboratory assessments, substance use and mental health evaluations, and social service needs intake, the patient was linked to a primary care physician, typically in the HIV clinic. If care was desired in a general medicine setting, then a primary care appointment was made in that setting, if possible with a physician the patient had seen in the DEU clinic. The latter was the case for Lamar, because although he was unwilling to change his substance use behavior at that time, he was willing to establish ongoing medical care in primary care. He agreed that I, a 37-year-old white male, would be acceptable as his physician.

Lamar taught me many invaluable lessons about how to care for an individual with HIV infection and a person with addiction. Here are two of the most important ones.

Lesson 1: Engage the Patient

Engaging the patient in medical care is of primary importance in caring for the HIV-infected and/or the substance-using patient in ongoing care. If you cannot engage an individual in care, then the potential benefits of medical care and any wisdom of the medical team will be only theoretical. Engaging is not having the patient agree to do what you recommend but rather having him or her be willing to discuss options. That means showing up. This insight was realized before the era of serious attention being given to the HIV Care Cascade (the HIV care continuum), which acknowledges the central importance of engagement in medical care. Over time, Lamar bonded with the DEU nurse and gained trust incrementally with me, his primary care physician.

Lesson 2: Listen to the Patient

Listening to the patient and being a physician willing to accept rejection of a medical recommendation for care is another key lesson. The era of shared decision-making had not arrived in the early and mid-1990s. Certainly shared decision-making about an approach to one's addiction was not in vogue in the United States. It is probably safe to say that shared decision-making was not a mainstay of clinical HIV care in that period.

The reality was that Lamar and I disagreed on many things when it came to what he needed to do to improve his health. Although he understood the need to change his substance-using ways, he was not willing to get help for his heroin addiction and injection drug use. He was unwilling to consider AZT (monotherapy at that time) for his HIV infection, as he said that "Everyone I know who went on AZT died. That AZT kills patients." As for our discussions concerning addressing his injection drug use, he did not like what he saw among his friends on methadone for opioid dependence: "I would rather use heroin, Doc." Despite our disagreements that lasted for years, he did see the wisdom of never sharing his injection equipment and using clean "works"—the paraphernalia employed to prepare and administer heroin.

Over time, these discussions evolved and became informed by experience, both Lamar's and mine. After serving some time in prison, upon release Lamar decided that the time was right to give up heroin for good. He agreed to enter a methadone treatment program to pursue that goal. He made that transition and remained in recovery, one day at a time, for over a decade. He transitioned off the methadone almost a decade ago.

He became exceedingly busy and sought-after for his skills in the auto mechanics trade. This work passion was a major resource for his recovery and positive outlook on life. This progress continued despite his ongoing long-term relationship with his female partner, who continued to use multiple substances. Despite the risk, which we discussed, that his girlfriend's active substance use posed to his recovery, he remained for decades in a committed relationship and in solid recovery.

Heart to HAART

The era of highly active antiretroviral therapy (HAART) came, and our discussions about the value of his considering this treatment became more frequent. Lamar had rejected any consideration of HIV medications for almost a decade, but an opening for reconsideration seemed to exist. His CD4 T cell count continued to trend down. He noticed that although people taking AZT may have died, those taking "the cocktail" were not dying. He said that he would "think about it."

In 2002 he agreed to start on HAART, and his response was excellent. His highly organized life worked in his favor with regard to effectively taking his medications. His avoidance all those years of HIV monotherapy probably was beneficial as far as his not having resistance to his HIV medications. His own decision to reject my recommendations years earlier, based on the collective wisdom of the medical establishment, was in retrospect the wise approach. He always appreciated our discussions on these topics and that we could agree to disagree; and in the end, his decision about his care trumped conflicting medical advice.

Who Would Have Thought

Recently, I told him that I was thinking about writing about his journey as an important aspect of my journey in understanding and learning to care for individuals who have HIV infection and had used drugs. He was honored. He said, "I would like that. You can use my name." He just retired from his work after almost two decades of often working 60-hour weeks. He remains on HAART with an undetectable HIV viral load. His spirits are very positive. His recovery remains strong. He has in the past year ended his long-term relationship with his partner, who was never able to achieve recovery from her substance use. He is fully engaged in medical care, but now in his sixties, he is very fit and not particularly medically complicated.

Who would have thought in the early 1990s, seeing a middle-aged man with an incurable deadly viral infection with an even greater life-threatening heroin addiction, socially stressed, and with serious legal problems, that a 2016 routine medical appointment follow-up would be so uncomplicated? Not me!

Unmoored

CHARLES VAN DER HORST

O NE EVENING IN EARLY SPRING 1980 during my medical internship, I
picked up a new admission in the emergency room of North Central
Bronx Hospital. Already on a ventilator, his lungs were filled with the fluid
of a diffuse pneumonia. No friends nor family were with him. Because he
was intubated immediately on arrival, we could not take an adequate history as to whether or not he had any chronic medical problems. He was
cachectic and looked like a survivor from a Nazi concentration camp or an
African famine. In places, his skin sagged, loose with soft folds, all his fat
and muscle consumed by his unknown disease. The rounded ends of his
bones pushed against his pale epidermis, tent-pole-like protuberances that
kept the skin lucent and taut. He was tied to his hospital bed, sedated, and
oblivious to his own suffering. The bones of his ribs protruding, the concave
hollowness of his abdomen, and the tilt of his head gave him a Christ-like
appearance.

The elevator moved up to the 10th-floor intensive care unit as I slowly
squeezed the football-shaped, rubber ball pushing oxygen-enriched air into
his lungs 15 times each minute. The ER chart provided no clues as to what
was causing his pneumonia. Reaching the ICU, the nurses and I hoisted him
into his bed. He lay beneath an unobstructed view of the blue sky and a
block print portrait of a figure with red lips and a big black fur hat, a tan-
gled spaghetti of tubes and wires snaking from his still body.

Despite my having a medical degree, the realities of internship were as far
removed from my knowledge and capabilities as a medical student as reading *The Art of War* is from bullets whizzing by your helmet and your buddy
keeling over dead next to you. At the start of internship, you go through the

motions of providing care even though you believe you are completely incompetent. You follow orders, start IVs, draw blood, take histories, listen to hearts and lungs, and struggle to maintain your concentration and focus, hoping that at some point, with repetition, you will achieve clarity and possibly even competence.

With six to eight admissions every three days and new problems and diagnoses to work up, I gradually became a more proficient physician. The routine tasks of listening to patients' chief complaint, eliciting their symptoms, and carefully looking for clues on the examination of all their organs and orifices helped guide my thoughts and inform my thinking about what process or disease was driving their problem. After a few weeks of internship, I began to develop the ability to create a mental list of the possible diagnoses or differential diagnosis immediately upon hearing the patient's first words, refine that list as I asked questions to elucidate factors that might lead the answer in one direction or another, refined further with lab test results, until through a process of logic and elimination, the one true answer would appear.

Despite the increasing sensation of competence as the year progressed, patient deaths, inevitable in a busy referral hospital and even expected, were like a cut inflicted on my soul, a symbol of my personal failure. The accumulation of unending small wounds took its toll.

Suppressing the doubts, I turned my attention to my new patient and proceeded to conduct a careful examination, reviewed his initial test results obtained in the emergency room, and ordered more tests. Through the gurgling of the tubing in his trachea, I could hear wet whispering diffusely in his chest. The inside of his cheeks were filled with a thick white coating. Neither his liver nor his spleen were palpable, and his heart sounds were normal. Around his rectum was a large ulceration, bigger than my hand, raw, red and moist. On his skin were scattered purple papules.

This constellation of physical exam findings, I quickly realized, was beyond my experience as an intern. I had taken care of many ICU patients by that time, but they all had single diseases despite many symptoms, fulfilling Ockham's razor or *lex parsimoniae*, the law of parsimony, a problem-solving principle that states that among competing solutions, the one that can cause all of the presenting signs and symptoms should be selected. My prior ICU patients had meningitis, pulmonary edema, severe asthma, septic shock with the blue fingers of hypotension, a gastric ulcer pumping blood out of the patient, or the crushing chest pain of a myocardial infarction. This person had multiple unknown lesions on his skin, a coating in his mouth, a diffuse pneumonia, and had wasted away. My threadlike feeling of competence and organization bumped up against his presentation.

The ICU in this hospital operated as an open system; that is, the ward teams, two interns and a resident, followed their patients from the floor to the ICU if they deteriorated and back to the general ward if they improved. By following the patients for 36 hours after their admission in the general ward or the ICU and then returning the next morning, I usually received instant feedback and satisfaction as my patients improved with my interventions: dilating airways in asthma, lowering glucose with insulin, killing bacteria with antibiotics. The feeling of gratification when I made the correct diagnosis and the macho joy of a successful treatment was infectious as the patients laughed with relief at their improvement.

As I looked through the floor-to-ceiling glass door, the chest of my unconscious patient rose and fell in a pas de deux with the white bellows of the ventilator. The whoosh of air in the tubing, beeps of IV machines, and the harsh guttural suctioning to remove thick mucus filled the silence. I was used to elderly people with unknown diseases, but a 24-year-old? I stared at him, stretched out and pinned to the bed, pale under the harsh fluorescent lights above and the light box on the wall. His chest X-ray revealed fluffy cotton shadows that overlay the white curved bones of his ribs, air spaces drowning in fluid.

To diagnose the etiology of a pneumonia, the first step is staining sputum to look for bacteria. Disconnecting his breathing tube from the ventilator, I snaked a clear plastic tube down his tracheal airway to suction any pus from his lungs. Unlike usual pneumonias, there was no green or yellow pus, only a white froth. Staining it for bacteria showed none, nor was there any fungus visible under a potassium hydroxide drop, a much rarer cause of pneumonia. After a negative stain for the bacteria that causes tuberculosis, I called the pulmonary fellow to ask him to perform a bronchoscopy to obtain a biopsy of the lung. This clearly was not a usual community-acquired pneumonia.

The weeping, beefy ulcer spreading from his anus to his buttocks was new to me, looking like the worst herpes lesion ever. The dermatology team came to look at it and the purple lesions on his skin and to biopsy each of them. His laboratory data revealed that he was anemic but he also had a low platelet count, and almost no lymphocytes, one of the white blood cells that fight infections. This is seen with patients on powerful chemotherapy drugs. But he was not on chemotherapy nor any other medicine that we knew of. I did a bone marrow biopsy and sent the specimen to the pathologist to look for the progenitor cells of the red and white blood cells and mega-karyocytes that produce platelets. Did he have malignant cells filling his bone marrow and displacing his normal cells, or was it an infection? Nothing explained his laboratory findings.

The test results and consultations dribbled back, each one adding to my bewilderment. The silver stain of the biopsy of the lung showed the black dots of *Pneumocystis,* a rare form of pneumonia seen in transplant recipients and chemotherapy patients. One of the first outbreaks of this pneumonia was seen in children who had survived the Nazi concentration camps.

The stain of the large ulcer revealed multinucleated giant cells, large pink cells at the surface of the skin with more than one purple nucleus, consistent with either herpes simplex virus or varicella zoster virus. The coating in the mouth was a fungus, *Candida albicans*, with transparent narrow tubular tangles, like Medusa's head, glistening in the light of the microscope. The stain of the purple papules on his skin showed elongated spindly cells with oblong purple nuclei and lakes of bright red blood cells in rudimentary vessels, consistent with Kaposi's sarcoma, a rare cancer usually seen in elderly men from the Mediterranean. Too many diagnoses, but I made my list of next steps.

On the wall of one of the hospital rooms was a series of small paintings. Each showed the inside of an airplane window looking out at the cumulus clouds and azure sky. This was a perspective I rarely had and certainly not with this patient. I was in the weeds and trees with no time to rise above to understand the big picture. I had read about Kaposi's sarcoma and *Pneumocystis* and seen herpes simplex, but not like this and not all at one time. No established treatment existed for Kaposi's sarcoma, nor were there any approved antiviral drugs for cutaneous herpes simplex. The only known treatment for his pneumonia was a toxic drug given intravenously, pentamidine, which was only available by calling the Centers for Disease Control (CDC) in Atlanta. The young CDC physician officer took my patient's history and told me he would arrange to ship the pentamidine. Just before hanging up he mentioned that there had been several other requests for pentamidine recently, which was highly unusual.

Despite my efforts, the patient's disease was too advanced. Supported by the ventilator, he was unmoored from anyone who cared for him, an unknown. Who was he? Where were his friends, his family? In the end, the boxes were checked off, the diagnoses made, and I was left with the frustration of not understanding why and watching this young man die alone, away from his family, with just the nurse and me holding his hands.

Postscript

June 5, 1981, *Morbidity and Mortality Weekly Report, Pneumocystis* Pneumonia—Los Angeles:

In the period October 1980–May 1981, 5 young men, all active homosexuals, were treated for biopsy-confirmed *Pneumocystis carinii* pneumonia at 3 different hospitals in Los Angeles, California. Two of the patients died. All 5 patients had laboratory-confirmed previous or current cytomegalovirus (CMV) infection and candidal mucosal infection. Case reports of these patients follow.

Yet Another Stigma
HIV Strikes People with Severe Mental Illness

FRANCINE COURNOS

YOUR PATIENT HAS AIDS, and there's nothing more we can do for her, so we're transferring her back to you." It was 1983 and the message came from Kings County Hospital, a huge municipal facility in Brooklyn, New York, known for its outstanding trauma care, heroic public health deeds, chaotic conditions, and occasional acts of unfathomable neglect. The message recipient was Kingsboro Psychiatric Center, an underfunded and chronically troubled state hospital for people with the most severe forms of mental illness.

The patient was a 25-year-old single white woman with severe mental illness and *Pneumocystis* pneumonia. In the absence of any other explanation, her pulmonary condition led to the diagnosis of AIDS. At that time, the responsible virus was called HTLV-III. There was no antibody test for it, and no understanding of how it was transmitted. Panicked staff, dressed in gowns and masks as if preparing for a moon walk, reluctantly approached patients. Hospital aides left food trays outside patients' doors.

Kingsboro Psychiatric Center was reluctant to take the patient back and asked for advice from its supervising authority, the New York City Regional Office of the New York State Office of Mental Health (NYSOMH). I was the chief medical officer, so it was my problem to solve. My first thought was that a dying woman with a terrifying infection didn't belong in a psychiatric hospital. That might have been a valid medical position, but Kingsboro was also the patient's home. She had lived there for the past two years, too psychiatrically ill to be discharged to a lower level of care. Going home to die was the norm for people with AIDS. Fortunately, Kingboro's medical director saw no problem with taking the patient home, so back she went to Kingsboro.

I was there the day she arrived, standing in a crowd of staff and administrators, watching as the medical director approached her. She held the patient's hand as she welcomed her back. This small act felt jarring, as if the internist had just put her hand into fire, and it served as a rebuke and a reminder that we hadn't entered the health professions to cower in fear.

Over the next few years in New York City, other patients in state hospitals would present with AIDS. Often we recorded their symptoms in their medical records without arriving at a diagnosis—a low white blood cell count, thrombocytopenic purpura, swollen lymph nodes, chronic diarrhea. It was only when they became dramatically ill that we would diagnose AIDS. At that point, few of our patients lived long and we provided hospice care. Staff members were dying too, mostly young male doctors and nurses who were closeted about their sexual orientation. They often disappeared without an acknowledgement of what had happened. Even now, I try to avoid mentioning the names of staff members who died of AIDS. If they went to the grave with a secret, who am I to violate their privacy?

Medicine Meets Humility

Early in the epidemic, the words of my medical school professors at New York University in the late 1960s kept coming to mind: "The one thing we have accomplished in medicine is the triumph over infectious diseases." A new epidemic caused by an undiscovered microbe was until now beyond our imagination. We had forgotten humility.

Gradually, the basics of managing the illness in our state psychiatric hospitals fell into place. In 1985, HIV antibody testing became available, and in 1986, following the first household contact study clarifying transmission routes, we instituted universal precautions. We learned how to give prophylaxis against opportunistic infections, and anxiously waited to see if agents might be developed to treat HIV itself.[1,2]

The leadership of the NYSOMH approached the spread of HIV infection among its patients largely by ignoring it. Maybe our state capital, Albany, was too far from New York City to feel the intensity of the epidemic. Maybe NYSOMH, like every other underfunded public agency, was not looking for more trouble. "Don't you want to know how our patients are getting infected, and how prevalent this virus is?" I would ask at meetings in our main Albany office. Silence was the answer.

Moving Past the Dichotomy

People with severe mental illnesses like schizophrenia and bipolar disorder die young, as much as 25 years earlier than the general population, mostly of medical conditions like cardiovascular and pulmonary diseases. Our healthcare system not only ignores this problem, but actively contributes to it. In medical settings, people who behave in unusual ways are often dismissed, avoided, stigmatized or feared, even when they pose no danger to others and are in grave danger themselves. And in psychiatric settings, where clinicians are trained to accurately observe and effectively respond to the ways their patients struggle with very real and debilitating psychiatric symptoms, there is minimal access to good medical care. Someone with a serious disease of the mind and also one of the body does not fit well into a system that declares the mind and body to be separate domains. Mounting an adequate response to the HIV epidemic would require moving past this dichotomy.

Treating Mind and Body

For most of my career I directed the Washington Heights Community Service, a program in northern Manhattan for people with severe mental illness, part of the New York State Psychiatric Institute and the Columbia University Medical Center. We had 22 acute inpatient beds and two outpatient clinics, with a combined census of about 1,000 patients, mostly recent immigrants from the Dominican Republic.

In 1988, we treated a 27-year-old single Dominican man with bipolar disorder and AIDS whose sexual behavior was too unsafe to allow for discharge. Long-term healthcare facilities would not take him—too mentally ill. Long-term psychiatric facilities rejected him—too medically ill. We were prepared to continue in a hospice role on our acute care inpatient unit. But then, remarkably, he was accepted at a newly opened residential program for AIDS patients in lower Manhattan. Despite having neither psychiatric nor medical services on site, this program did not consider our patient too mentally ill or too physically ill to be transferred there, underscoring the fear and stigma that had led to his being rejected for admission by the more traditional institutions to which we had initially turned.

The residential program was in a building originally designed as a luxury hotel for gay men. Patients' rooms were beautifully furnished and had panoramic views of the Hudson River. Ironically, our patient spent his final months living in the most beautiful home he had ever known. This resolution presaged the migration of people with severe mental illness and HIV infection out of the psychiatric system and into the specialized HIV/AIDS care system for all of their services.

Making Research Headway

By this time, I had given up hope that NYSOMH would ever investigate any aspect of the HIV epidemic among its patients. In 1989, with the help of Karen McKinnon, Anke Ehrhardt, and other colleagues at New York State Psychiatric Institute and elsewhere, I obtained a grant from the National Institute of Mental Health to study rates of HIV infection and HIV-related risk behaviors among the patients in my own program and at Creedmoor Psychiatric Center in Queens, where my good friend and fellow psychiatrist Maureen Empfield served as clinical director.

Our study found that among 451 consecutively admitted inpatients anonymously tested for HIV-1 antibodies from December 1989 through July 1990, the prevalence of HIV infection was 5.5 percent, with comparable rates in men and women.[3] Black patients accounted for only 38.0 percent of the patients tested but 76.0 percent of positive HIV test results, a rate of 11.1 percent for this group. Infection control records suggested that clinicians were aware of only 7 (28.0 percent) of the HIV-positive cases, indicating our system was largely failing to identify them. The fact that 1 in every 18 patients admitted to two state psychiatric hospitals in New York City was HIV positive was startling.

We also interviewed people with severe mental illness to gain a better understanding of how they had become infected. At a governor's reception in Albany where I took the opportunity to advocate for better sexual health services in state psychiatric hospitals, the response of the legislators I spoke with was largely incredulity: "What? Psychiatric patients have sex?" I couldn't effectively counter their disbelief because, in fact, we knew very little about the sexual lives of people with severe mental illness.

So we conducted intensive interviews with 178 of our psychiatric patients. Among the 52 percent who were sexually active in the past 6 months, there was considerable high-risk behavior: 48 percent had multiple sex partners; 35 percent used drugs during sex; 30 percent traded sex for drugs, money, or other goods; and 58 percent never used condoms.[4] Trading sex was more than three times as likely among patients with schizophrenia as among those with other diagnoses. In addition to sexual risks, 18 percent of patients had a history of injection drug use. All this despite the fact that patients were generally well informed about AIDS.

No one from the NYSOMH Central Office contacted me to discuss any aspect of these findings, and eventually I asked why. "Take that as a message" was the response. Those of us concerned with the HIV epidemic in psychiatric patients were mostly on our own.

An Integrated Treatment Approach

Over the years, as it became possible to live with HIV infection, people with severe mental illness and HIV infection increasingly migrated out of the mental health system and into the HIV care system. And, surprisingly, patients with illnesses like schizophrenia seemed to have an easier time accepting HIV infection than previously healthy people who became infected. Our patients were already familiar with having a stigmatized illness requiring ongoing treatment with medications that had unpleasant side effects. In a sense, HIV was just another problem, another stigma, piled on top of a life of struggle.

Multiple studies conducted worldwide have repeatedly confirmed that psychiatric patients have elevated rates of HIV infection. Studies in the United States suggest a 6 percent HIV infection rate among people with severe mental illness, with similar rates in men and women.[5] This may be an overestimate, given the concentration of studies in the severely impacted Northeast region, but nonetheless it is more than 10 times higher than the general US population. When patterns of HIV-related risk activity are compared with the general population, a higher proportion of people with severe mental illness have a recent history of sexual abstinence, but those who are sexually active have elevated rates of risk, including multiple sex partners, men having sex with men, buying or selling sex, and injection drug use.

Time and medical advances have done little to change the response of NYSOMH to HIV infection. For example, while HIV testing is now universally recommended in all US healthcare settings, NYSOMH has exempted itself from carrying out this mandate in its own psychiatric hospitals.

Perhaps it's easier to integrate the care of the mind into the medical system than to integrate the care of the entire rest of the body into the psychiatric system. Perhaps those who choose to work with patients with a stigmatized medical condition like HIV infection find it hypocritical to reject people who have other stigmatized problems, like mental illness. But one thing that we have definitely learned in this epidemic is that there is no clear division between physical and mental illnesses, and only an integrated treatment approach is plausible.

References

1. Cournos F, Empfield M, Horwath E, Kramer M. The management of HIV infection in state psychiatric hospitals. Hosp Community Psychiatry 1989 Feb;40(2):153–7.

2. Horwath E, Kramer M, Cournos F, Empfield M, Gewirtz G. Clinical presentations of AIDS and HIV infection in state psychiatric facilities. Hosp Community Psychiatry 1989;40(5):502–6.

3. Cournos F, Empfield M, Horwath E, McKinnon K, Meyer I, Schrage H et al. HIV seroprevalence among patients admitted to two psychiatric hospitals. Am J Psychiatry 1991;148(9):1225–30.

4. Cournos F, Guido JR, Coomaraswamy S, Meyer-Bahlburg H, Sugden R, Horwath E. Sexual activity and risk of HIV infection among patients with schizophrenia. Am J Psychiatry 1994;151(2):228–32.

5. Cournos F, McKinnon K. HIV seroprevalence among people with severe mental illness in the United States: a critical review. Clin Psychol Rev. 1997; 17(3):259–269.

AIDS Case Management
A Community Response

GIBBIE HARRIS

IN THE MID-1980S, like many counties across the country, Wake County, North Carolina, was beginning to understand the multiple challenges the AIDS epidemic was presenting to the community. And like other communities, we were not prepared to support the individuals who had been infected with HIV. At that point in the epidemic, most of the individuals infected were young, gay men who had left the South to avoid discrimination. Now, ill with a disease that was not well understood, they were returning home in the hopes that their families and communities would care for them.

The predominant reaction to HIV in the South, and in Wake County, was fear and condemnation. Much of the fear was based on a lack of knowledge of the disease, the perceived risk of transmission, and the certain death that seemed to be the fate of those who were infected. The stigma that already existed toward gay men and that had caused them to leave their homes in the first place was heightened by the disease they were contracting. Some felt they deserved AIDS and that they had brought this on themselves with their "lifestyle."

For most people living with AIDS, their medical condition resulted in loss of jobs, loss of insurance coverage, loss of housing, and loss of their support system, including family and friends. Even churches that historically had supported their communities in times of difficulty hesitated or declined to get involved. For some it was a lack of understanding and education on the issue; for others it was a moral judgment of those most often infected.

The medical community and those who provided support services to those with chronic or fatal diseases also were challenged. There was little training available on how to diagnose and treat AIDS. Medications were nonexistent or limited to palliative treatment. And the possibility of transmission was considered an unacceptable risk for many healthcare workers. Hospitals were crowded with people living with AIDS who were often too ill to be discharged without a place to go and someone to care for them. Their care was costly and the lack of insurance coverage was straining the healthcare system.

In Wake County, the three county hospitals—Wake Medical Center, Rex Hospital, and Raleigh Community Hospital—were experiencing the strain and burden of beds filled with dying AIDS patients for extended periods. There was no cure, and very little in the way of treatment was available to slow the progress of the disease. Few medical providers would see these patients. There were no systems in place in the community to support people living with AIDS. The number of patients was growing and AIDS care was becoming quite taxing.

Efforts were under way in North Carolina to try to catch up with the effects of the epidemic, as it was already too late to get ahead of it. The NC Department of Health focused on policy development, the issue and availability of testing, discrimination, and the development of a system of care. Gay rights advocates and organizations were leading efforts to reduce discrimination and to support those already infected. The Wake County Department of Health was working hard to educate the community and keep fears tamped down, focusing on prevention, especially for those most at risk. They also provided contact tracing to identify those who had been exposed and to provide testing to them.

These were critical efforts in the fight to manage this disease, but care for those already ill also was needed. In addition, there was the challenge of individuals not willing to come forward for testing for fear of losing their jobs, insurance, and housing, especially when it seemed there was little or no healthcare to support them. This resulted in a growing hidden epidemic of a fatal disease that left its victims in a state of severe social, professional, and healthcare isolation.

Despite all of these factors, a handful of compassionate, dedicated advocates created an environment that led to the creation of one of the first AIDS case management programs in the South and the first in North Carolina. Three important efforts came together at the right time. First, the hospitals were searching for a solution. Second, a handful of churches stepped up to provide practical support. Third, and possibly most important, one individual, Sandy Hendrickson, a nurse who worked for the health department, had already emerged as an advocate and a volunteer care provider for people living with AIDS. Sandy knew the system well enough to manage it for the patient's benefit. She worked tirelessly, and with immeasurable personal power she was able to motivate others to help her in this effort. She already had the trust of people living with AIDS in the community.

The CEOs of the three hospitals came together with the Wake County health director to figure out how best to address the most critical issues they were facing. This led to the creation of the Wake County Hospital Alliance. Through contributions and the commitment of the four entities, they agreed to fund case management services to address the needs of AIDS patients. Initially, the program was funded with $350,000 from the Hospital Alliance. At that time, these hospitals were also paying insurance premiums for people living with AIDS to help cover some of the medical costs.

Although there was a great deal of mistrust on the part of people living with AIDS of government and even nonprofit agencies, the decision was made to create the program within the Wake County Department of Health. Support from the Wake County Board of Health and Wake County government to provide services for people living with AIDS was critical to the beginning of an organized AIDS case management program in North Carolina. However, it was very challenging to work around the "system" to build a system that could be trusted by those who were disenfranchised. It required responsive, brave, committed leadership; financial support from the hospitals and the Health Department; expertise in knowing what was needed; and having compassionate advocates to know how the system needed to be built.

Sandy Hendrickson was already working in the community with people living with AIDS, and she understood their needs and their fears. Consequently, she was able to bring others to this work in a way that was nonjudgmental and inclusive. In 1988, she was the architect for the AIDS Case Management Program. The Wake County Department of Health hired two nurses (including Sandy) and two social workers to begin providing services. They worked with others in the community to create the support system and to educate and advocate for tolerance and prevention.

The focus of the AIDS Case Management Program was on medication, access to care, and housing. A strong partnership with the AIDS Service Agency of Wake County, formed in 1991, was a critical next step in the development of housing opportunities and meeting the day-to-day needs of people living with AIDS. At this point in the epidemic, individuals did not survive long and case management was truly hospice case management. The emotional support provided by the case managers and the AIDS Service Agency staff was effective because of the trust developed with people living with AIDS.

Another example of the partnerships that made these efforts successful was the case managers' work with churches. A few congregations were already preparing frozen dinners to be delivered to those living alone and too ill or weak to cook for themselves. The case managers became the meal delivery system. This effort evolved into the Triangle AIDS Interfaith Network (TRAIN), which aimed to provide practical support to people living with AIDS. TRAIN eventually created care teams, based on a national care team model, to provide broader support to meet the increasing needs of community members. Case managers worked closely with the care teams, often making the original referrals to them. This weaving of services to create a safety net for people living with AIDS again exhibited what a community can accomplish when brought together under a unified goal.

A significant challenge facing the system of care was the discomfort of the medical community in providing care to people living with AIDS. It took a handful of brave physicians in Wake County and a strong connection with the University of North Carolina (UNC) AIDS Clinical Trials Unit to allow access to the care needed by people living with AIDS. These relationships led to the creation of a Ryan White clinic at the Department of Health in 1991. This clinic was made possible through US Human Resources and Services Administration funding provided through the local federally qualified health center, Wake Health Services; physician support through UNC; and Wake Medical Center support for inpatient care. The ongoing efforts of the AIDS case managers to link patients to care and support their lives in the community made this clinic successful.

The creation of the AIDS Case Management Program was motivated by the mission and drive of compassionate advocates. It took hard work and determination not to fail. However, complicated health and social issues require broad partnerships. They also require a system approach to encompass the total needs of the individuals and how to meet those needs. Working in isolation is rarely successful. Policies and programs needed to evolve to address the needs of this new health threat. Although there are any number of efforts these days that focus on social determinants and the need to purposefully address them if health improvements are to occur, this was not a well-described concept in 1988. Nonetheless, bright, creative people knew this intuitively and were able to come together to make a difference. Through leadership, financial support, and advocates unwilling to take no for an answer, the Wake County community made it happen when it was most needed.

AIDS care has evolved from treatment for a fatal disease to treating a chronic condition. However, the need for case management endures and has evolved to address the changing groups affected by this disease. For example, the long-term medications required to manage this now-chronic condition are costly and often hard to obtain. AIDS Case Management and Medication Assistance Programs are still there to assist. Through ongoing leadership, effective partnerships, and strong advocacy, Wake County still strives to meet the needs of people living with HIV/AIDS in the community.

Acknowledgment

Many thanks for the input and memories from Steve Cline, Jacquelyn Clymore, Leah Devlin, and Yvonne Torres.

Women and Pioneering Women

Cherchez la Femme

Yes, the French Woman Did It.
She Discovered the AIDS Virus.

MARY GUINAN

D R. FRANÇOISE BARRÉ-SINOUSSI at the Institut Pasteur in Paris was responsible. I knew it, others knew it, and of course she knew it. But someone else loudly proclaimed that he had done it. And he was a world-renowned scientist at the National Institutes of Health (NIH), powerful, brilliant, and so convincing that the scientific community believed him, despite the evidence that was always there.

Those of us who worked at the Centers for Disease Control (CDC), where the AIDS epidemic was discovered in the 1980s, still wonder why she remained so quiet amid the outrageous claims of the NIH scientists and the lawsuits and counterclaims of French scientists.

The Nobel Prize, a dream of many scientists, was on the line. Her name was rarely, if ever, mentioned. After all she was French, an unknown junior scientist, and a woman. How could she and her colleagues have scooped Dr. Robert Gallo and the NIH? And she almost got away with being anonymous. That is, until 25 years later, when she, along with her colleague, Luc Montagnier, won the 2008 Nobel Prize in Physiology or Medicine for discovery of human immunodeficiency virus (HIV), the AIDS virus.

Why did it take so long for Françoise Barré-Sinoussi to be recognized? She was, after all, the first author of the 1983 article that reported the discovery in *Science*, one of the most prestigious medical journals in the world.[1] All scientists know the importance of being the first author of a scientific research paper because it indicates the person who did the major part of the work.

What happened during those intervening 25 years turned out to be one of the most incredible scandals in the history of medical research. NIH scientists claimed the discovery of the AIDS virus and ignored or dismissed the work of the French, all with the collusion of the US government. Much has been written of the scandal, including the results of the intensive multiyear investigation by John Crewdson, a Pulitzer Prize–winning journalist. In his 2002 book *Science Fictions: A Scientific Mystery, a Massive Cover-Up, and the Dark Legacy of Robert Gallo*, he describes how Gallo, at the National Cancer Institute at NIH, and his colleagues claimed to have discovered the AIDS virus and obtained a US patent for a blood test for it in 1985.[2] Subsequently, Gallo received worldwide acclaim and numerous prestigious awards, including a 1986 Lasker Award and a 1988 Japan Prize for his "discovery." Often, these awards are a prelude to the Nobel Prize in Medicine. But Gallo was wrong. He hadn't found the AIDS virus; the French had.

The French filed a series of lawsuits against the US government concerning these claims starting in 1985. When the evidence could no longer be suppressed, US government lawyers advised NIH to settle the case. In 1994, NIH finally acknowledged that Gallo had used the French virus for the blood test that he had patented and for which he and NIH had received the patent royalties. Future patent royalties would largely go to the French.

After the Nobel Prize in Medicine was awarded to Barré-Sinoussi and Montagnier, Crewdson noted on his website:

> Not included in that award was Robert Gallo, who for many of those
> 25 years had attempted to claim credit as the discoverer, and later the
> co-discoverer, of HIV. With that verdict, science at last accepted what
> the evidence had long shown, that the fundamental discoveries leading to
> the recognition of HIV as the cause of AIDS had occurred in France, and not
> in Gallo's laboratory at the U.S. National Cancer Institute. One of the most
> divisive and destructive disputes in modern scientific history had at last been
> laid to rest.[3]

Collective Amnesia

But has it? I often give lectures to public health workers and students on the history of the AIDS epidemic. In the eight years since the Nobel award, I always ask my audience, "Does anyone know who received the Nobel Prize for discovery of the AIDS virus?" As of 2016, not one person has known the name Françoise Barré-Sinoussi. Many thought it was Gallo. This common misperception is reinforced by profiles of Gallo in the media and on the Internet, including Wikipedia, that name Gallo as co-discoverer of HIV, without mentioning who the other co-discoverers were nor who actually received the Nobel award for the discovery.

I decided that I wanted to know more about this mystery scientist, Françoise Barré-Sinoussi, and hear her story. In summer 2014, she graciously accepted my request for an in-person interview at her office at the Institut Pasteur in Paris. My sister, who speaks French better than I do, accompanied me. But she spoke English beautifully, so we needn't have worried about language difficulties.

Background

The first report of five gay men with the syndrome we now know as AIDS appeared in 1981 in the *MMWR* (*Morbidity and Mortality Weekly Report*), CDC's weekly newsletter.[4] The article in the *MMWR*, which is sent to health authorities throughout the world, triggered a worldwide alert that something deadly was affecting gay men in Los Angeles, as two of the five men had died. Were there cases elsewhere? Did the disease only appear in the gay population? Who else was at risk for the disease? Were there cases in other cities or countries? Who, when, what, where, and how are basic questions that medical detectives had to answer. CDC created a task force of highly skilled medical epidemiologists, statisticians, and laboratory workers to investigate. I was one of 30 members of that first task force.

CDC is command-central for monitoring disease activity all over the world, especially new and deadly diseases. Within days, reports of cases came pouring into CDC from state and local health departments, hospitals, and physicians' offices; and, more slowly but consistently, from Europe and Africa. It was frightening. The death count was soaring and the cause of the disease was unknown. These case reports were compiled into surveillance data, which were reported in the *MMWR*. Eventually, analysis of these data showed that AIDS could be transmitted through sexual intercourse between both homosexual men and heterosexual men and women, among drug users who shared needles, from blood transfusions and blood products used for the treatment of hemophilia, and from affected mothers to their newborn infants.

These modes of transmission were exactly the same modes of transmission as those for hepatitis B virus. The evidence was clearly suggestive that the cause of AIDS was a transmissible agent, most likely a virus. However, despite extensive studies of blood and body fluids from hundreds of AIDS patients, a suspect virus was not found. The clinical clues from the accumulating surveillance data showed that whatever was causing the disease was killing a particular white blood cell, the T lymphocyte, which plays a central role in the body's immunity against disease. The cause of death for most

AIDS patients was an unprecedented breakdown of the body's vital immune system, which allowed all kinds of bacteria, viruses, fungi, parasites, and tumors to proliferate and suck the life from the patient.

If the cause were a virus, it was a new and deadly one. To virologists, the effect on the immune system suggested that the cause might be a retrovirus. The high-stakes race was on to find it. I and most scientists working in the field believed that the discovery of the virus would be followed soon by the development of an effective vaccine to prevent the disease and eventually eliminate it. We had reason to be optimistic. After all, smallpox, also a viral disease, had just recently been eliminated from the world with an effective vaccine and a dedicated worldwide effort. And it looked like polio, measles, and mumps viruses would eventually meet the same fate.

But it was critical to find the virus first. Neither a drug to cure AIDS nor a vaccine to prevent the disease could be developed without the virus. And AIDS was spreading at an unbelievably rapid pace. The longer it took to find the virus, the more it would silently spread around the world.

In 1983, after giving a lecture on AIDS to a medical audience, I was asked, "How long will it take after the discovery of the virus to develop an effective vaccine?" I replied naively, "From six months to a year." (I still have nightmares about seeing this exchange on YouTube.) How wrong I was! As of 2016, some 33 years after the discovery of HIV, an effective vaccine to prevent its transmission still eludes us.

Before the emergence of the AIDS epidemic, retroviruses had been shown to cause leukemia in animals, including feline leukemia. Such findings led to an intense search for a retrovirus as a cause for human leukemia. Most retroviral researchers were cancer specialists with little expertise in infectious diseases, including one of the most prominent, Robert Gallo at the Laboratory of Tumor Cell Biology at NIH, who had discovered the first human retrovirus, which he named HTLV.

In France in 1983, the Institut Pasteur in Paris was doing the most retroviral research, led by Luc Montagnier, Jean-Claude Chermann, and a junior scientist, Françoise Barré-Sinoussi. Clinicians in Paris had appealed to the Institut to help them investigate the cause of AIDS. Soon an extensive collaborative group was organized between the Institut and Parisian clinicians and virologists.

Françoise Barré-Sinoussi

As Dr. Barré-Sinoussi recounted her story to me, she credited Dr. Donna Mildvan, who was then chief of infectious diseases at Beth Israel Medical

Center in New York, for giving her the idea of looking for the virus in a lymph node. Mildvan had reported that, prior to developing AIDS, many gay men experienced a "diffuse persistent lymphadenopathy" or "lymphadenopathy syndrome" of unknown cause; that is, continuous swollen lymph nodes in different areas of the body, including neck, groin, and underarm. Perhaps lymphocytes in the lymph nodes were fighting the AIDS virus and had multiplied and swollen the lymph nodes.

No one had yet looked for the virus in a lymph node. On January 3, 1983, Barré-Sinoussi received the lymph node specimen she had requested, which had come from a patient with lymphadenopathy syndrome. At the Institut Pasteur, the specimen was put in a culture of T lymphocytes, a method developed by Gallo's NIH laboratory to grow retroviruses. Barré-Sinoussi and her collaborators agreed that she was to monitor the culture for growth and then test the fluid in the culture for an enzyme—reverse transcriptase—which is found only in retroviruses and is necessary for their reproduction. This was the definitive test for the presence of a retrovirus.

However, to her dismay, Barré-Sinoussi found that whatever was in the lymph node was not causing the T lymphocytes to grow but instead was destroying them, similar to how whatever was causing AIDS was destroying the T lymphocytes in human patients. And she was worried. If the virus was present, she had to keep it from dying—and the virus needed lymphocytes to keep from dying. She came up with the idea of adding more lymphocytes so the virus could keep reproducing. She acquired lymphocytes from the Institut blood bank and added them to the culture. If a retrovirus were in the culture, it needed T cells to reproduce and she had to increase the number of T lymphocytes reproducing so that the reverse transcriptase enzyme would increase to a level that could be detected by the test.

Every three days, she checked the culture. On January 23, 1983, she performed the radioactive test for reverse transcriptase on the culture fluid. The result was 7,000 counts per minute, indicating a small amount of reverse transcriptase. But three days later, she repeated the test and the result was 23,000 counts per minute. There was no doubt about this level. The team had found a human retrovirus, and it had to be a new one because it didn't act at all like Gallo's HTLV. The French team named it lymphadenopathy-associated virus, or LAV.

The team quickly began to write up its findings to submit to a medical journal. Because the premiere medical journals are in English, Barré-Sinoussi described to me how the team struggled to get the paper written in precise scientific English. I asked her if there was any question who would be the first author. She said, "No, because it was clear I had done the work."

Montagnier called Bob Gallo at NIH and asked for reagents from his laboratory. Gallo asked why. The answer was, "We have found a new retrovirus and we want to compare it with your HTLV." Gallo was very interested and told Montagnier that the journal *Science* would soon be publishing a special section on retroviruses for which Gallo himself was submitting several papers. Gallo promised that if the French team sent its article to him he would convince *Science* to include it in that issue. The French team rushed to complete the manuscript and sent it to Gallo.

However, in their rush, they had forgotten to include an abstract, the introductory part of a scientific paper that summarizes the content. An abstract is required by most medical journals. Gallo called Montagnier and said there was no time to wait for an abstract from them so he would help the team write it. Gallo wrote the abstract and called Montagnier on the phone and read it to him. There was something in it that Montagnier did not think was correct. It was the statement that LAV was likely part of the HTLV family of viruses. The French team knew it was not. But Gallo insisted on the wording and Montagnier finally relented.

Barré-Sinoussi did not see the abstract before publication. Montagnier later told her that agreeing to put that statement in the publication was the worst decision of his life. Later, Gallo claimed not only that he had found the AIDS virus, which he called HTLV3B, but also that he had isolated it in 1982, before the French did.

DNA to the Rescue

How was the question resolved? How was it proven that Gallo had used the French virus for his blood test? Viral DNA. Just as human DNA studies of a crime scene have implicated suspects and the lack of their DNA at the crime scene has cleared many others, HIV DNA pointed to the French as the true discovers of the AIDS virus.

As it turns out, HIV DNA is very variable. As more and more isolates of HIV were studied, it was remarkable how different their DNA and genomes were. No two are exactly alike. The virus keeps mutating, which is one reason why an effective vaccine has not yet been found. But when scientists compared the LAV used to make the French blood test with the HTLV3B used for the NIH blood test, it turned out that the DNA and genome were almost identical and *had to have come from the same patient*. It was a French patient. How ironic that the virus provided the proof.

I asked Barré-Sinoussi why she had kept such a low profile during the fight for the recognition of who discovered the virus. She replied that she was a laboratory scientist and she had never worked with patients. At that time, she was working with a team of physicians and virologists who were desperate to find something to treat patients with AIDS. Patients often joined the team meetings. When the controversy between the French and American scientists became public, the patients at one of the team meetings accused the team of only caring about who got the credit for discovery of the virus and not about the patients. She decided at that point to focus her energies on how to help the patients and to stay out of the fight.

The Institut Pasteur started looking for drugs that might control the virus. The team did a series of trials on possibly effective drugs. In fact, many Americans went to France to participate in these trials, including the famous actor Rock Hudson, because there were no ongoing treatment trials in the United States.

In addition to her laboratory work, Barré-Sinoussi became involved in education programs for developing countries on how to prevent HIV infection and in getting HIV antiviral medications to even the poorest countries. She worked with Francophone countries, such as Vietnam and Cambodia, and became a prevention activist. She told me that she felt it was a compliment to be called an activist.

I asked her if she had known that she was possibly "on the list" for a Nobel Prize. She said she had no idea. In fact, she was in Cambodia at a meeting when the Nobel Prize winners were announced. The Nobel Prize committee couldn't find her, and she had not been told of the award before the winners' names were released to the media. On the morning of the announcement she received a call from a friend who worked for French radio. The friend was crying, and Barré-Sinoussi asked what was wrong. The friend was saying something about the Nobel Prize but she couldn't understand her. She said, "I will call you back because I am at a meeting," and turned off her phone. But the phones of many at the meeting were ringing, and her colleagues told her she must answer her phone. The Nobel Prize committee finally located her.

She celebrated that evening with colleagues at the French Embassy. And then she had to go back home. When she arrived in Paris very early in the morning, she heard a great commotion when she got off the plane but couldn't see what was going on. As she walked into the airport, she heard a great roar. It was a crowd of people from her laboratory and others cheering with flowers and placards congratulating her.

I asked Barré-Sinoussi if she thought others should have been included in the Nobel award. "Yes," she said, "I think that the award should have gone to the team rather than just the two individuals." She specifically named one

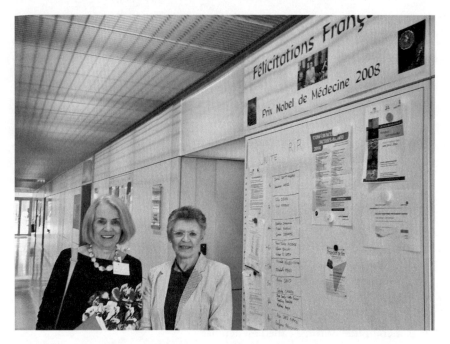

FIGURE 6.1. Dr. Mary Guinan (*left*) with Dr. Françoise Barré-Sinoussi at her laboratory at the Institut Pasteur in Paris, May 2014. Photo courtesy of Mary Guinan.

of the coauthors of the publication, Françoise Vezinet-Brun, for her very important contributions.

Barré-Sinoussi has published more than 200 papers advancing the knowledge of retroviruses, and her advocacy role for the prevention and control of HIV infection is exemplary. She has used her stature as a Nobel laureate to advocate for programs to bring HIV treatment and prevention programs to the neediest countries. She even called out Pope Benedict XVI when on his first visit to Africa in 2009 he told the press that the use of condoms only made the HIV/AIDS epidemic worse. She sent the Pope an open letter that stated that he should know better. He had access to the best experts in the world to learn about the effectiveness of condoms, and his words to the press were not true. She told him what harmful effect his words would have on the HIV/AIDS-prevention efforts in Africa, a continent ravaged by HIV, and asked him to reverse his position. What a woman!

"You had such courage," I said. "Well," she replied, "I had to do something. The Pope has such a powerful voice on the African continent." Then she said sadly, "The Pope never responded."

References

1. Barré-Sinoussi F, Chermann JC, Rey F, Nugeyre MT, Chamaret S, Gruest J et al. Isolation of a T-lymphotropic retrovirus from a patient at risk for acquired immune deficiency syndrome (AIDS). Science 1983;220(4599):868–71.

2. Crewdson J. Science fictions: a scientific mystery, a massive cover-up, and the dark legacy of Robert Gallo. Boston, MA: Little, Brown; 2002. Originally published in a Back Bay paperback edition; 2001.

3. Crewdson J. Science fictions [book sales website]. Retrieved May 4, 2017, from http://www.sciencefictions.net/

4. Centers for Disease Control (CDC). *Pneumocystis* pneumonia—Los Angeles. MMWR Morb Mortal Wkly Rep. 1981;30(21):1–3.

The Needlestick Accident That Launched Healthcare Worker Safety

A Nurse's HIV Journey

LYNDA ARNOLD

I WAS BORN IN ROSEMONT, Pennsylvania, the oldest of five girls and the first child to go to college in my family. It was a big deal. After attending Catholic University, I went to York College of Pennsylvania to study nursing. I felt a real sense of accomplishment when I graduated with a BSN.

I interned in the emergency room at the Community Hospital of Lancaster. When I graduated, they were opening the intensive care unit. New nurses typically don't start in the ICU, but because I had emergency room experience, and they knew me, once I passed my boards they were happy to hire me into the ICU. I felt honored to be working there, and it challenged me physically, spiritually, emotionally and, most importantly, intellectually. I enjoyed the comradery of the respiratory therapists, the physicians, and of course the nurses. I was inspired by how the nurses did their jobs and how they dealt with very challenging and sometimes horrible situations. I knew then that I wanted to be a critical care nurse. I loved everything about it, even my 3:00 to 11:00 p.m. shift.

Accidents Happen

On September 9, 1992, we received a patient into the ICU who was a direct admit from his doctor. Although that meant he bypassed the ER, he still needed some IV lines placed so that we could treat him with fluids and any IV medication that the physician might prescribe. I set out to care for him like any other patient. We found out through a verbal report that this patient had AIDS.

I was aware of AIDS in Lancaster County in 1992. I knew how it could be transmitted, but I wasn't scared of contracting HIV. That said, I hadn't encountered anyone with the disease. Well, I probably had treated patients with it, but didn't know. We knew from the physician's office that this patient had AIDS and that essentially he had "come home to die." Cases like this were not uncommon in the 1990s.

My job was to start the IV line on him. When I decided where I wanted to insert a big bore needle into his arm, I chose an 18-gauge needle. I wore my gloves, cleaned the area, stuck the needle in his arm after I got a good placement, got a flash, and pulled the needle out. While pulling the needle out, he moved his arm up and hit my hand that held the needle. It went straight into my left palm, through my glove, into a jagged-shaped tear. I yelled for help and my supervisor came in. I said, "Jeff, I just got stuck. I need you to hold him down for me so I can tape him up." He said, "I'll tape him up for you. Go wash your hands. Take your gloves off. Right now, go wash your hands." That's what I did. Jeff finished taping him up and he said, "You need to go down to the ER and report this. There are forms for it." I got the forms, filled them out, and turned them in. Nothing else was done except for testing, because at that time there was no prophylactic regimen like PrEP. All we did was report what happened.

The next day, employee health started the testing and surveillance process. I hadn't heard of any doctors or nurses being infected with HIV in this way, so I figured I was going to be fine. I started the testing that night. Then employee health went through the protocol. I was tested at baseline, 6 weeks, 3 months, and 6 months. My baseline came back negative. I did not have HIV at the time of the needlestick injury.

The patient died 10 days later, which we now know meant his viral load was probably very high, but we didn't test for viral load then. I was feeling fine. I don't recall having any flu-like illness during my seroconversion. Up until month six, I tested negative. Somewhere between month three and month six, I seroconverted.

In the months between the needlestick and testing positive, I was still working in the ICU and trying to live a normal life. I was in my early twenties. I had met this guy named Tony and we started dating. He was in the Air Force and stationed at Dover, Delaware, about two and a half hours away. I had told him about the needlestick injury, but he didn't know anything about HIV or AIDS. We didn't really talk much about it.

When I got the call on April 7, 1993 to stop by the employee health office, I knew there was trouble as soon as I opened the door and saw worry written all over the secretary's face. I went into the room with the employee health nurse. I don't remember hearing the words "You have HIV" but I'm pretty sure she said them several times. I do remember sitting there thinking,

"I want to die. No, I don't want to die. But how did this happen? People are going to hate me. My life is over. I can't face all the discrimination. I'm going to have such stigma attached to me. Will people throw rocks at my window? Will people try to blow up my car?" These thoughts raced through my head simultaneously.

Then she started asking about my sexual partners. I told her about Tony. Then she said, "Anyone before?" I said "there was someone before that I saw for a little while." She said they both had to be tested immediately. There was a notification process and we went through it. I said, "I have to tell Tony tonight." He had just asked me to marry him, and now I had HIV!

I was so confused and the world around me was spinning and chaotic. I felt like I couldn't breathe. When I got home, I called Tony. I just remember crying and telling him, "I'm so sorry. I'm so sorry. We never should have gotten together. I didn't know." He didn't let me talk much. He just drove up immediately. Both of my sexual partners tested negative.

I also had to tell my parents, which was really hard. I had become independent. I had graduated from college. I had this great job. I was doing really well, and now I had to say, "Oh, my god, I screwed up." Even though the patient moved, in my mind with my parents, I had messed up. When I called my mom and dad that night, they were in shock. I don't think I had even told them about the needlestick. They had a lot of questions, some of which I couldn't answer. They wanted to come see me. Tony had also called his parents, who I had never met. It was Easter weekend and they wanted to come down for Easter, so both sets of parents were coming. I don't remember much about that weekend, but somehow we got through it.

I started telling my friends. People didn't understand how you could get HIV, so there was a lot of stigma. I decided it was better for me if I just told everyone because I'm not good at keeping secrets. Eventually I went public.

The first three years of living with my infection are a blur. Tony and I got married on May 13, 1994. I was hospitalized a lot because of the side effects of the medication. I had hepatitis, liver issues, meningitis, pancreatitis, neuropathy, fungus infections, and yeast infections, and my hair fell out. I couldn't tolerate any of the drugs that they used to treat HIV in the early days.

Tony got out of the military on an honorable discharge because he told his commanding officer about my health status, although I wish now that he had stayed in. We didn't know then what we know now about the virus, and about my medical needs, and about the military changes. We just knew what we had in front of us and we had to make a decision. So he got out and worked three jobs for a while to support us. I was working on and off at the hospital and sometimes receiving workers' compensation. In 1993, the hospital removed me from direct patient care and placed me in quality assurance. Then I had to be more on workers' comp because of the side effects of the drugs.

I found a good network of people and I got involved with the Lancaster AIDS project. I began to do speaking engagements—and then I found my best friend, Steve Foresman. Steve was about 10 or 15 years older and he had been infected that much longer. He was an inspiration.

I joined the support group for HIV-positive people in Lancaster. Although I felt I had found a home, I also felt like a spy, because if you look at me and you don't see HIV it's because I'm not who you think might typically get HIV. I just did not fit the "profile."

I became an active volunteer for the Lancaster AIDS Project. Steve and I used to tag-team and do speaking engagements all over the county in high schools, churches, and businesses. Often people didn't want to bring a gay person into their buildings or into their communities. But interestingly, they would accept me as a heterosexual female, along with this gay man. Maybe because in some way I made the presentation cleaner, nicer, or more presentable.

The Campaign

In 1996, I decided to launch a national campaign for healthcare worker safety because I found out through the employee health nurse at the hospital that there were somewhat protected needles—where either a sheath comes over them, or the needle retracts, or it's spring activated—or needleless systems that connect into IV tubing. All kinds of options for blood draws.

Our hospital actually had those needles for an IV line insertion, but they hadn't been put on the shelf yet. On the day of my needlestick, they were still stored in the basement. Once I knew about those needles, and that they hadn't even gotten on the shelves, it angered me and I felt unsafe for myself and for my fellow healthcare workers.

I began thinking about how many other needlestick injuries may have occurred and I started to research it. I met a doctor and three other nurses who had been infected with HIV through occupational exposure. I decided to create a campaign for healthcare worker safety to prevent these types of injuries. This meant I had to go public with my story.

I tried to get pledges from hospitals nationwide to implement these safer needle devices. We got a lot of publicity on TV, film, video documentary, newspapers, print, and elsewhere. I met many good people who care about this issue. I traveled around the country and the world with this campaign for healthcare worker safety. Prevention of accidental needlesticks had support from the unions and the American Nurses Association, and it took on a life of its own.

When I initially started the campaign, it was simply a movement to get healthcare organizations—specifically hospitals across the country—to sign a pledge that they would use safer needle devices, such as needleless IV systems, spring-based injection systems, protective IV catheters where the sheath comes over them, or phlebotomy devices where the sheath comes over or you pulled back the sheath to activate it. Because I was so adamant about the use of these devices by healthcare systems, I decided to go public. In going public, we got a lot of support across the country and I got a lot of support for the campaign.

So much so that I was able to make it into a 501(c)(3) organization. We put my husband at the helm as the president of the organization. He would filter out the requests and help organize and coordinate the activities, because one of the key things was that I was being invited to speak all over the country to healthcare workers at annual meetings or conventions, for example. My schedule needed to be coordinated and my husband was great at that.

At that point, I was on and off workers' compensation. I was generally committed to running the campaign for healthcare worker safety. I was primarily on workers' comp so I wasn't working a side job. I would get a stipend for my time, but I wasn't really making any money.

The campaign lasted from 1996 to 2000. I hit almost every state in the country except Alaska and Hawaii, and the furthest away it took me was Durban, South Africa. In 2000, the Federal Needlestick Safety and Prevention Act passed. That was really a culminating moment for me and felt like a huge accomplishment in my life.

In that regard, having HIV has been a blessing because had I not been positive, had I not been the second healthcare worker in the state of Pennsylvania to contract HIV occupationally, I don't think I ever would have started the healthcare worker safety campaign. Had I not had the experience as a child of watching activism and knowing what activism was, I don't think I would have ever started anything like that.

Memory Issues

Around 9/11, I started having issues with my memory, attention to detail and concentrating, which was becoming problematic at work as dosages and math were never my strong suit. Getting patients' medications right was extremely complicated for me, especially when I had more one than one or two patients. I started to see a neurologist and after conducting tests they found that I had mild neurocognitive disorder.

I applied for Social Security disability, and I told workers' comp that I wanted to go on permanent workers' comp disability. So I had a general review for that and I was approved for both Social Security disability and permanent workers' comp. Obviously, our income took a big hit. We moved to California where I had a good provider and family support.

If I had had a crystal ball and knew I'd be living with this virus for as long as I have been—and all the life changes, and problems, and consequences that have come from living with HIV—I might see things very differently now. But above all else, Tony was my best friend, and I love him very much, and I know that he loves me very much. However, there were always problems in our marriage—financial, sexual, dealing with the stigma, dealing with the secrecy, deciding who to tell, when to tell, who could know, who couldn't know.

I also had to deal with my own feelings of guilt, shame, and embarrassment. They call it survivor syndrome. I didn't have a lot friends that I lost to AIDS. One friend from the Lancaster support group got sick and died. I met people along the way that I'm sure are no longer with us. But I traveled in and out of so many different circles that I wasn't always necessarily with large groups of people living with HIV. I was pretty mainstream, and I had a diverse group of people at my side most of the time.

Regarding the campaign for healthcare worker safety, I had a lot of ammunition because the device manufactures, the unions, the American Nurses Association, and the Service Employees International Union quickly got behind me. Though my dream of having every hospital in the United States sign the pledge to protect their healthcare workers by using safer needle devices seemed like a lofty one, I didn't know how relatively easy it would be.

I also didn't realize what a big business this was and what all this really meant. I just didn't want someone else to get infected like I had been infected. That's really what my story is about. But over the years, it morphed into my story from the needlestick injury. I'm grateful that I could use that medium to get my story across, and that it really helped a lot of people. I wouldn't say I'm thankful for having the virus, but I'm grateful that the virus allowed me to touch so many lives, and to effect change on a national level.

Also, at the time we were in litigation against the needle manufacturer. We ended up settling out of court, but I wouldn't say that we used our money wisely. I mean, we did buy a house, and we have since moved a lot, and we traveled some, and we saved some, and we blew a lot of it because we were young and stupid. But we didn't really save for a rainy day because we didn't think that rainy day was coming; at least I was never convinced that it was.

Medically, in the first 10 years of my infection, everything that went wrong with me had very little to do with HIV per se, but had everything to do with the medications. I was either allergic or too sensitive to almost every drug and drug combination they gave me. I was either sick with a rash, or hives, or horrible diarrhea, or vomiting. I would end up hospitalized with drug-induced hepatitis or meningitis or pancreatitis. That's when I began to really feel the effects of my neuropathy.

It wasn't until after I had gotten out of the campaign for healthcare worker safety, had stopped working for the needle manufactures, and had gone back into staff education and agency nursing that I began to sense the mental slowing. I was losing my place in my calculations, for example, or I was aware that it was taking me three or four times longer in multiple-step calculations. I realized this wasn't safe and that it was unfair to my patients.

That's when I had my first battery of psychological tests in which they identified neurocognitive difficulties. The psychiatrist explained that it was like driving over a bridge, looking back, and not remembering how you got there. That was a spot-on description.

I was also under a lot of stress and my depression became evident. I had been depressed before. I'm sure I had depression as a child or a teenager, actually; especially having been sexually molested. But for the first time in my adult life, it was really evident. I was very, very blue. I got rid of almost anything of meaning to me when we moved from Pennsylvania to New Jersey, because we were moving into a smaller house. I just didn't care. I was very apathetic.

I had a hard time during that transition. We were forced to face bankruptcy, which was sad. I thought we had made smart decisions regarding finances and real estate, but we hadn't. We had overextended ourselves. So a running theme through my life became apparent: highs and lows, money issues, spending habits, and then the faltering depressions. I just lived that way and functioned at that level. But in 2007, I was awarded full disability for the rest of my life and I went on Social Security disability.

Stigma

I've now been living with HIV for over 22 years, and as the years go by it becomes harder and harder to get a doctor to accept workers' comp. Each time I have to explain how in the world I have HIV workers' comp for a gynecological, pulmonary, dental, cardiac, or bone density appointment. It's literally gotten to the point that we've had to split my medical care between two different facilities because it's so complicated.

I have Medicare now, secondary to my HIV workers' comp, but also secondary to my primary insurance that my husband carries. Every day I get bills that are overdue, aren't paid, or threaten me for collection. But they're not my responsibility. They're the responsibility of workers' comp, but the hospitals don't bill correctly. So I face stigma and discrimination every day in the healthcare system.

Also, from the beginning, I've had doctors on television and in person say, "Oh, she must not have known what she was doing. Oh, that poor girl. They put her right into the ICU. She never should have been in the ICU." Or, "Oh, she must not have been wearing her gloves." Or, "Oh, her technique was incorrect." No, that's not true. I knew what I was doing. I was a good fit for the ICU. I wore my gloves. I took my time. I followed proper procedures. It just happened. Accidents happen.

At the time I was injured, nearly 1 in 250 people in the country were known to be HIV positive. Over 800,000 needlesticks occurred annually. I never thought I'd be that 1 in 250. I never thought I'd be one of those 800,000 needlestick injuries.

The stigma and discrimination that I faced, and continue to face, is one of disbelief or of pity. When it comes to discrimination, I would say it's about paying my medical bills. The arguments between Medicare, my private insurance, and workers' comp, including my pharmaceuticals, center on who's going to pay and where that pay source is coming from. It has become more difficult and challenging day after day, year after year.

Adherence

Another issue that's challenged me is a common theme for many people living with HIV: adherence to medication. I adhered to my medication when I wanted to. When I wanted to get pregnant, I was extremely adherent. My viral load was undetectable. My T-cell count was terrific. I didn't do anything to screw up that pregnancy. I was a smoker. I stopped smoking. I did everything right. I ate right. I did everything I could to make sure that baby was healthy. But when it came time to take care of me, I wasn't so diligent.

Early in my treatment I was adherent, and I got burned by it. I had so many problems and side effects with the drugs it just tore me up. It would take me hours to take my HIV medicine. I would stare at it and move my pills around. I couldn't take it. I had a psychological block to taking the pills, primarily because of my stress and the trauma of having taken the pills and experiencing bad side effects, which would always land me in the hospital or the ER.

Even though the medications were getting better and the side effects were fewer or less severe, for some reason I couldn't wrap my mind around that. I was on and off my medication when I needed to be on it all the time. When I finally did crack and had that depressive break, we sold our house and moved to New Jersey, and moved away from the area that our kids had grown up in and loved. We had built that new house and I was back working full time at two jobs. Tony was teaching and life was just beautiful and chaotic at the same time . . . and depressing as much as it was happy.

I was miserable. As it turned out, I was having cognitive issues, which were discovered by a psychologist. I wasn't adhering to my medication. If I had been adhering to my medication, I may not have gotten those early cognitive problems. But the early cognitive problems really set me off because it made me afraid of what could happen. It made me value my husband and my kids so much more. I realized how much I had missed of their growing up with all of my travel, my work, my volunteerism, and my activism. Because of that, I was really shaken up and depressed. Instead of taking pride in all the work that I had accomplished, I wanted it to all go away. I wanted to go back to the beginning. I wanted to start over. And I no longer felt safe. I felt like my life was out of control and I needed something to grab onto.

Ultimately, we sold our house in New Jersey and moved to Los Angeles. But I was still nonadherent to my medication. I didn't think anything bad was going to happen. From what I figured, "Well, I'll take it when I get sick" or, "I'll take it later when I really need it." I had this nurse practitioner and I nearly always showed up for my appointments. They also had a psychiatrist, a nutritionist, and a dentist. I did everything right that way. Sometimes I would lie and say I was taking my medication. Other times I told her the truth; that I couldn't take them or I wasn't taking them. It was a good couple years we lived in Los Angeles until things really started to go wrong.

Coming to California was like an escape and I got to start over. It was the one time that we told the kids, "Okay. Let's not talk about HIV." Because I wanted normalcy. I wanted my kids to grow up without the shadow of HIV surrounding them. So we all agreed that's what we were going to do. That's what I told everybody, "Just leave me alone. I want to raise my children. I don't want to be in the spotlight. I just want to have a normal life."

Everybody from the community respected that, from journalists to hospital workers to the researchers to the unions. I really appreciated that. I threw myself into volunteering with a talent management firm. A couple years in, my oldest had some issues with school and with the law, and I had a breakdown at that time. I wasn't taking my medication, and I didn't put two and two together.

I thought I was just stressed about my son's activities. Looking back, I can say that I wasn't on my meds, and had I been on my meds I probably would have handled things better. I probably would have been able to recuperate more quickly. The breakdown came and went and things moved on again.

A couple of years later, still not adhering to my medication, we again had some issues with my son, and I had another type of breakdown. I blamed it all on situational stress. I didn't see the pattern in "you're not taking your medication. Something's going wrong here." Once again, we got my son the help he needed, and I pulled it together and organized everything for the family, because that's my role.

Somewhere in there, I lost myself. Those cognitive issues that I had back when my son was about four had now escalated. At this point, he was 16 or 17. Those issues escalated, which changed my life forever.

I was admitted to a psych hospital in Los Angeles for three weeks. It was horrible. The people were nice. The staff were great. But the mere fact that I was in a psych hospital was "crazy." I was diagnosed with HIV dementia—it's probably one of the most stigmatizing diagnoses that anyone can get—and being HIV bipolar. I don't remember much about the actual hospitalization, except we did of lot of arts and crafts, and group therapy sessions. Even in my group sessions they cautioned me not to talk about HIV, which I thought was strange, but I went along with it. They were unsure how the other patients would respond. So I always skirted around it. I talked about my brain and my brain issues. I never brought up HIV the whole time I was there.

Finally, somebody gave me a referral and we got to a new HIV doctor. I went into the UCLA system, and I met Dr. Ardis Moe. The first time I met with Dr. Moe, she told me, "You're not going to die from HIV." And I thought, "Okay, that's good to know." She put me back on a regimen of HIV medication that was very difficult for me to take. I only stayed on that regimen for a short period, when she said, "Okay, we'll stay off it." So she tried keeping me off it, like I had tried all those years. She said, "When you're ready, we'll get back on it."

Well, I got really sick. We decided to put in a feeding tube so that I could get the medicine through the tube and I wouldn't have to swallow it. Apparently, that had worked for other patients. It was a good idea except for the fact that the tube got infected, and then my immune system was so compromised that I got septic throughout my whole body, and I nearly died. I was in the hospital for more than 60 days. I had to go to rehab. I was on TPN (total parenteral nutrition, a method of feeding that bypasses the gastrointestinal tract). It was horrible.

My T-cell count dropped to something like 42, which is the lowest it had ever been. Slowly, very slowly, I began to pull out of this abyss. I was on Neupogen, which I had to inject twice weekly. I had a hematologist. We had to do bone marrow biopsies and spinal taps. That period of my life, from 2012 to 2014, was a medical nightmare. It was so horrible because they were trying to get me back on track. If not, I was going to die. I didn't want to die, but I also didn't want all these horrible treatments. About that time, things finally started to calm down and we were able to get the right medication, at the right dosage, and medicines that I wasn't allergic to.

Between 2014 and 2016 my health has stabilized. The one thing that has continued to be a huge problem has been the neurocognitive issue. In the past year I've suffered horrendous memory loss, and my brain (and my body) has aged more rapidly than the brains of my peers. It's gotten particularly worse over the past year. Some is long-term memory loss. Some is short-term. Sometimes I can't remember things that happen in the same day. It's really scary for me because I feel it's progressive.

Right now, I'm at the point of trying to stop some of my insular medication that could be causing my memory loss. We're going to be going to the Memory and Aging Center at the University of California, San Francisco, to try and figure out what's happening. I've been through all different kinds of psychological and neuropsychological testing at UCLA three or four times now, and the diagnosis of HIV dementia and neurocognitive impairment still sticks.

I'm also about to start treatment with ketamine, which is IV, for pain and depression. Once we can lift the pain and depression, before we go to the Memory and Aging Center, I'm hopeful that they'll be able to pinpoint the cause of the memory loss because some of the drugs I use for pain and depression can cause memory loss. If I can get off those drugs, then hopefully we can find the true culprit causing the memory loss.

The Future

I don't know if I'm going live to be 75 or 85. I know HIV is considered a chronic, long-term condition now. I'm trying really hard to be adherent to my medication, and I'm doing a good job. My viral load is undetectable. My

T cells are at the low end. They're hanging in there around 300, which is good for me. Right now, my stomach is cooperating. I've had some cardiac issues this year, which they blame on the HIV. But my workers' comp carrier doesn't believe HIV causes cardiac issues, so we have that over with my regular medical doctor and medical insurance.

I definitely have had some pulmonary issues this year. Once again, workers' comp doesn't believe HIV causes pulmonary issues. So that's with my regular medical team. But these have been my main problems related to HIV: my stomach, my heart, my lungs, my eyes, my brain, and my skin. I try to keep a cheery outlook. I try not to complain every day. I know that my husband thinks I complain every day, but I could complain more.

I go to counseling every week. Other than that, I try to enjoy my life. I went on a cruise this year for people with HIV and their partners or their spouses, but I had to go alone because my husband had to work. I met a lot of great people, many of whom are long-term survivors like me.

I think the future of addressing HIV rests in people like me, long-term survivors, and figuring out how we're still here, and how the virus has attacked the body over the years. But it also lies in the prevention of new cases. Working at the AIDS Project of Los Angeles, I see so many new cases. It's really sad. I don't understand where we've gone wrong with the lack of education. We should have conquered AIDS by now.

Yes, we need a cure. Yes, we need a vaccine. Yes, we need support for people living with HIV. But what I mostly get upset about is when I hear people talk about HIV as if it's just, "Oh, I take one pill a day and I'm fine." You know, for some people that works and that's great. But for a lot of people, like me, one pill a day doesn't work.

My hope for the future is that we eradicate HIV from the planet. And that people wise up and realize that once we get rid of HIV, there's likely to be another bug lurking around the corner. So we have to put into play all of the things we learned from HIV—have safer sex; use condoms; eradicate drug use, especially injection drug use and needle sharing; eliminate domestic violence; eradicate poverty; teach at the point where lessons are needed most, eat well and exercise; and solve homelessness to name a few.

I feel that we made the hospital and healthcare system safer, but it's not 100 percent. People have to activate the devices a lot of the time, wear their gloves, and use common sense.

My story was never just about HIV. It's about living with a disability. My goal as a survivor is to help others not become HIV positive, and to help those that are living with HIV to live full and happy lives. There were so many people that helped us along our journey. Not just our family, not just our immediate friends, but people whose names I don't remember. People whose faces I've forgotten.

If my memory could be counted on, I would be able to say thank you to all those people individually. But I can't; it's all gone. When I look at pictures now, it doesn't help to bring back specific memories. Yet there are indelible imprints on my heart and that can't be taken away. No loss of memory is going to take the inference off my heart. That I know.

HIV is not who I am, but it is a part of who I am. At times it's a very big part of who I am. Do I think HIV is going to kill me? No. I think Dr. Moe is right. I'll die of something. We all do. Will I have to fight HIV until I die? Hopefully not, but maybe.

This is my story. I'm still living day by day, making each day count, living my life to the fullest, making my share of mistakes, trying to learn from them, trying to treat the problems that exist, hoping, and creating new memories along the way, even if they're only imprinted on my heart.

HIV Takes Center Stage

MARY JANE ROTHERAM-BORUS

INITIALLY, MY WORK IN HIV was driven by academic politics, not personal interest. Only after I was publicly committed and conducting HIV research did issues emerge among my extended family that cemented my interest and led to a 30-year commitment to the HIV field. Without a salient personal or family issue, I doubt I could have sustained my HIV work. My story also reflects how work issues can reverberate within one's life to take center stage.

In 1987, as a professor of child psychiatry at Columbia University in New York City, I was interested in school-based prevention research, mainly aimed at social skills deficits in young children. Having moved from Los Angeles to New York City for my husband four years earlier, I was living a hectic life with stepchildren, a biological daughter, and a daily 20-mile commute into New York City. I was busy. Since coming to Columbia University, I had worked with suicidal youth and homeless youth, the primary interests of the Division of Child Psychiatry at Columbia University at the time.

HIV emerged on the public health radar in 1981. However, it had not been a highly salient issue to most traditional departments of psychiatry. The primary populations affected by HIV were gay and bisexual men, hemophiliacs, and injecting drug users. Young people, especially homeless youth, were at risk, but no one knew how at risk. Additionally, no preventive intervention studies had yet been conducted. The best the field was mounting were epidemiological studies that showed that a generation of gay men, hemophiliacs, and injecting drug users was going to be decimated, quickly and with rapid declines, and horrible symptoms such as going blind, getting uncontrollable fungi, and becoming paralyzed. I had known a few faculty who had tested seropositive for HIV, but it did feel salient to my life.

In fall 1986, while a professor at Columbia University, Anke Ehrhardt led a review team for the National Institute of Mental Health (NIMH) to evaluate if the University of California, San Francisco, should receive a federally funded center to promote research on HIV prevention. She returned confident that Columbia University could also receive funding for a similar center. As a member of the department who worked with populations at risk HIV infection, I was recruited to lead a preventive intervention project for homeless and gay/bisexual youth. My project was to be one of two projects for adolescents: one on high-risk youth, headed by me, and one on school-based prevention, headed by Heather Walters. Studies of disease progression complemented our prevention studies, as well as epidemiological studies of sexual risk. We organized a program project application and submitted it to the NIMH in spring 1987, with a site visit scheduled to review the application on June 22 of that year. We rehearsed and were prepared for this site visit and felt confident we would wow the reviewers.

On June 12, 1987, my husband died suddenly of a heart attack. I was given a week to get back to work.

The reviewers came, the entire team did well, and we were funded. We encouraged the team to go to Times Square to watch on the central news-feed billboard the announcement of a $20 million HIV prevention center granted to Columbia University.

Researchers mobilized, research teams were built, and a set of cutting-edge studies on HIV prevention, disease progression, and epidemiology proceeded. HIV research became the dominant area of my academic life. I had two cohorts of young people to recruit, interventions to design and evaluate, a husband to grieve, and children to support during their grief. Needless to say, this was a busy and stressful time.

At the same moment, my cousin living in Hawaii called me. She had HIV, as did her husband. Her two children, 4 and 8 years old, were uninfected. She needed help and wanted me to tell the family she was infected.

My cousin had been a star as a child and adolescent: smart, beautiful, athletically talented, and warm. She was a regional medal winner for swimming. As a graduation gift from high school, she went to Hawaii for vacation. She never came home. She lived on multiple islands, became involved with a surfer peer group, and became an active drug user. She and her husband were HIV infected. Her partner was incarcerated, right before she called me for help. My personal and my professional lives were aligning to face similar challenges.

I am the oldest of 12 cousins, all of whom grew up in the Los Angeles area and 10 of whom still lived there. I was in New York and my youngest cousin was on the Big Island of Hawaii. I visited her in Hawaii. She lived in a home on a rural dirt road, and it took her an hour a day to take her children to their school bus stop or to deliver her trash to a junkyard. I helped her move to a new apartment in a small city-type setting, on the beach. Taking out the trash became a two-minute activity daily, rather than a half-day or full-day process.

Visiting my cousin's family alerted me to the kinds of issues I would see in my intervention research. In 1993, I was funded to conduct interventions for families living with HIV.[1-13] This funding occurred concurrently with an exacerbation in my cousin's symptoms. Her children had not been told that their mother had HIV, yet, the children accompanied their mother and me to the Big Island AIDS Project. AIDS information was posted on every wall of the center. We talked about AIDS in the children's presence. We talked about the fears about AIDS. She was taking medication and had multiple side effects. My cousin complained about her husband (still in jail). These were daily conversations, but she believed the children did not know that their mother was HIV positive. This came to be a key finding in the research I later conducted with families living with HIV. Mothers with AIDS (not HIV, but AIDS) who had adolescent children claimed their children did not know about their illness. Yet in their homes, there were pamphlets about AIDS, medications for HIV, friends with AIDS visiting, and hospitalizations for AIDS in rooms that could only be entered with facemasks and full-body coverings. The children did not know (or claimed not to know) their parents' serostatus.

My cousin expected to make it for the cure. I was leading pilot intervention groups in New York City with mothers with AIDS in 1993. The Department of AIDS Services only served mothers with a diagnosis of AIDS. When we started our project, the official registry of the Department of AIDS Services consistently showed us that time to death was 14.9 months. I would be conducting a group with women who had their head fully bandaged from the neurosurgery they had the previous week. They were in wheelchairs and could barely talk. Nonetheless, these women believed they would make it for the cure. I would sit in the room and hope no one died while we were conducting the group. The amazing fact is that more than 60 percent of the women did make it to the cure. Six years later, after the efficacy of AZT and shortly after that the introduction of antiretroviral therapy (ART), more than 60 percent of the mothers who had been expected to die in 14.9 months were still alive.

HIV mobilized many mothers to get their lives together—to stop using drugs, to eat better, to be spiritually healthier, and to sleep in regular routines.

Almost all mothers (86 percent) in our New York City cohort had been heavily involved with drugs. Yet there had been dramatic reductions in substance use when learning of their HIV status. Not only did mothers reduce their use, they moved from injection drug use and heroin to less lethal types of substances, such as alcohol and marijuana. My cousin gave up injection drug use and heroin when she learned her serostatus.

Depression was rampant among mothers with AIDS. About 30 percent reported specific symptoms that a full diagnostic interview would have indicated meant a depressive disorder. Depression, rather than HIV, was often the more debilitating and challenging disorder for these women. My cousin died because of depression, not because of HIV. Many years after her children had left home, she killed herself. Her death was related to anger, anxiety, and depression because of her life circumstances, not HIV.

I saw the similar challenges among injection drug users in Vietnam, who are highly stigmatized. Yet, families will never abandon a family member with a drug abuse problem, as the family will be shamed and the injection drug user will have no social status or possibility of getting a job or recovering. It is the stigma that can lead recovering addicts, who have also acquired HIV, to kill themselves prematurely. Their death frees their families from stigma and themselves from a marginalized life. Today, the US president's strategy and the Office of AIDS Research has prioritized comorbid conditions as those that must be addressed to eliminate HIV. Comorbid mental health and substance use conditions have been ongoing challenges from the beginning of the HIV epidemic.

My cousin's children lived with me for about 10 years. They were adolescents before I knew them well. I had successfully mounted and demonstrated substantial and significant improvements among both mothers with AIDS and their adolescents over six years of follow-up prior to having my cousin's children live with me. The adolescents in our research study had lower rates of substance use, were more likely to graduate from high school, were less depressed, and had fewer babies as adolescents, and their babies tended to have better homes and higher IQs. These were pretty impressive outcomes. During breaks in the intervention group meetings, adolescents would tell me, "We are learning not to act out our feelings. We are taking better care of ourselves."

Yet, when I tried the same activities at home with my cousin's children, I was refused: "Forget it, Mary Jane. I am not doing these things. I do not want to talk about my mother. Go away." Maybe if my cousin's children had had access to a program mounted by someone outside their family they might have been more receptive to the intervention. I could not even get these children to role play, or to talk about fears or depressed thoughts. I wonder whether the evidence-based interventions are better delivered at a later age, not during adolescence.

In designing the intervention, I had anticipated that it is at the time of significant life events that children are most affected by the loss of loved ones. My cousin's oldest daughter is getting married in a month. I have never seen her so happy with a partner, so in love, and so committed. She has planned this event for more than a year. She has no ambivalence about the partner. But she called about a month ago and for the first time in her life she was interested and started a conversation about her mother. She could not understand why she was feeling depressed. She is so in love and happy with her life. How or why is she depressed?

Her experience matches most of the literature on children who lose parents. Now is the moment when her mother is missed the most. Her mother would be going with her for the fitting of the wedding dress. Her mother would wear a dress the color of her bridesmaids. Her mother would be hosting the rehearsal dinner. Her mother would be giving a toast. I am not there for her now, but I will be at the wedding. We talk often. She is living in Hawaii and I do not live there. The most significant relationship she has ever had is missing at one of the happiest times of her life.

When I was beginning my research, "Memory Boxes" were being used all over Africa. There was no data to support their use, and there is none today, although the fad has passed and I do not believe that the use of these boxes remains. Every clinical program I knew about in the 1990s was getting mothers to make videos for their children. We tried this with our intervention studies. We were totally unsuccessful and had no positive examples to share from trying to get mothers to make videos. We did not distribute the videos made by the mothers to their children. Among at least 30 videotapes, there was not a single mother who did not wag her finger at her son or daughter, reminding them, "I told you to . . . if you are in trouble, you obviously have not done what I told you to do."

My cousin did not leave her children a Memory Box or a video. Hopefully, her final phone calls are not remembered. Yet every remembrance of my cousin is valued by her children, daily. I can trace their preferences in clothes, hair styles, and lifestyle to her influence. Their childrearing practices are similar to their mother's best childrearing practices.

My cousin's oldest daughter, now in her early thirties, is old enough, free, and independent enough to mourn her mother. She can appreciate how much her mother gave to her each day when she was young. She knows what it means to be a mother 24 hours a day. As she prepares to become a mother herself, the loss of her mother is heightened. I expect at every major life event, the loss of a loved one is reexperienced. It is the long-term consequences of HIV that our research is not designed to assess.

When I was working with families, I found three families in which the mother had HIV and her adolescent child also had acquired the virus. The *New England Journal of Medicine* pointed out the possibilities before I saw my first case. While the cases can be seen as reflecting children immersed in the lifestyle of their parents, such as injection drug use networks, there appeared to be other dynamics in each case. Only in the context of seeing young people with their parents repeatedly over time did I observe the unfinished issues of the parents. Children who had not obtained the approval and unconditional love of their parents may seek this love in self-destructive ways. Parents who derailed their own lives with drug use often berate their children for following in their footsteps. The consistent haranguing of the children appeared to result in the enactment of the parents' worst fears. In each case in which the children became HIV infected, the parents' admonitions appeared to result in the children doing the opposite of what their parents advised, but almost exactly the same as their parents' behaviors.

Nearly all prevention programs, and even clinical psychotherapeutic interventions, address challenges at the behavioral level. Yet, repeated behaviors over time become predictable habits of daily living, themes that characterize a life, and unresolved conflicts that can dominate the psychological life of children as they become adults. HIV infection among children of parents with HIV is an area in which these themes emerge repeatedly. In the future, these issues must be addressed within communities and families.

HIV was not my life's passion; children and families are my passion. But I have been able to integrate my passion into the issues that are most salient to HIV. In the past 10 years, I have opened family wellness centers in low- and middle-income communities. I am hoping to initiate these changes in communities devastated by HIV. I have been working in South Africa and Uganda, two countries in which children and families have been affected. My work has always addressed concurrent health challenges of malnutrition, mental health, and alcohol and other drug use. However, I have written extensively about the importance of prosocial, community-level, structural interventions. Family wellness centers could be the preventive supports needed and a vehicle for evidence-based interventions to be mounted nationally and globally. It is to this mission that I commit the remainder of my career.

HIV has provided me with a vision and purpose for my career for the past 30 years, and it has repeatedly intersected with the challenges faced by my own family. In Africa, very few families are untouched by HIV. In America, many families have gay and bisexual relatives whose lives are affected by HIV. New pandemics are emerging. In the next 10 years, the Zika virus and hepatitis C are far more likely to influence American families. Yet these epidemics create the opportunities that have been present throughout the ages. Our work becomes a vehicle to connect us to others, inspire us, and increase our humanity. Alternatively, it can lead us in the pursuit of personal aggrandizement, accumulation of accolades, and a disconnection from others. My cousin and her children inspired me not to succumb to be only a driven researcher in a cocoon, lacking the empathy that these real-world challenges require.

References

1. Rotheram-Borus MJ, Stein JA, Lin YY. Impact of parent death and an intervention on the adjustment of adolescents whose parents have HIV/AIDS. J Consult Clin Psychol 2001;69(5):763–73.

2. Rotheram-Borus MJ, Lee MB, Gwadz M, Draimin B. An intervention for parents with AIDS and their adolescent children. Am J Public Health. 2001; 91(8):1294–302.

3. Rotheram-Borus MJ, Leonard NR, Lightfoot M, Franzke LH, Tottenham N, Lee S-J. Picking up the pieces: caregivers of adolescents bereaved by parental AIDS. Clin Child Psychol Psychiatry 2002;7(1):115–124.

4. Rotheram-Borus MJ, Lester P, Wang PW, Shen Q. Custody plans among parents living with human immunodeficiency virus infection. Arch Pediatr Adolesc Med 2004;158(4):327–32.

5. Rotheram-Borus MJ, Flannery D, Lester P, Rice E. Prevention for HIV-positive families. J Acquir Immune Defic Syndr. 2004;37 Suppl 2:S133–4.

6. Rotheram-Borus MJ, Lee M, Lin YY, Lester P. Six-year intervention outcomes for adolescent children of parents with the human immunodeficiency virus. Arch Pediatr Adolesc Med. 2004;158(8):742–8.

7. Rotheram-Borus MJ, Flannery D, Rice E, Lester P. Families living with HIV. AIDS Care 2005;17(8):978–87.

8. Rotheram-Borus MJ, Weiss R, Alber S, Lester P. Adolescent adjustment before and after HIV-related parental death. J Consult Clin Psychol 2005; 73(2):221–8.

9. Rotheram-Borus MJ, Lester P, Song J, Lin YY, Leonard NR, Beckwith L, et al. Intergenerational benefits of family-based HIV interventions. J Consult Clin Psychol 2006;74(3):622–7.

10. Lester P, Rotheram-Borus MJ, Lee SJ, Comulada S, Cantwell S, Wu N, Lin YY. Rates and predictors of anxiety and depressive disorders in adolescents of parents with HIV. Vulnerable Children and Youth Studies 2006;1(1):81–101.

11. Rotheram-Borus MJ, Stein JA, Lester P. Adolescent adjustment over six years in HIV-affected families. J Adolesc Health. 2006;39(2):174–82.

12. Rotheram-Borus MJ, Swendeman D, Flannery D. Evidence based family wellness interventions, still not HIV prevention: reply to Collins. AIDS Behav 2009;13(3):420–3.

13. Rotheram-Borus MJ, Swendeman D, Chovnick G. The past, present, and future of HIV prevention: integrating behavioral, biomedical, and structural intervention strategies for the next generation of HIV prevention. Annu Rev Clin Psychol 2009;5:143–67.

"Don't Die of Ignorance"
A Scramble for Knowledge

LORRAINE SHERR

ONCE UPON A TIME—a game-changing time, a scary time, a riveting time—a long time ago a new virus emerged. An exceptional virus, a retrovirus, a global virus blind to borders and groups. Rarely are we present at a point in history—a crinkle in time—where something changes and it is irreversible. We all ask, where were you when Kennedy was shot? Where were you when planes hurtled into the World Trade Center on 9/11? Where were you in the '60s? But more importantly for this tale, where were you in the '80s? The giddy moments when the lengthy-named human T-lymphotropic retrovirus, or HTLV-III virus, was stutteringly discussed, in harmony with LAV (lymphadenopathy-associated virus) and the political decision to rename it HIV.

My story starts at this moment. By a curious coincidence, I was based at St. Mary's Hospital in London—the hospital with the largest sexually transmitted infections clinic in Europe. I was training to be a clinical psychologist and my training was rudely interrupted. I delivered my baby on the day of my final qualification examination with the British Psychological Society. Although I negotiated (difficult in those days) discharge from hospital within hours to drive up to Leicester for my examination, the British Psychological Society examining board ruled that if I arrived late I would not be examined (remember, they are the caring profession). The effect of that decision fed into my curious coincidence. I had to postpone my final examinations and qualification. I took my maternity leave in California, where my husband taught at UCLA, and I wrote my PhD thesis under the boardwalk, on a blanket, with a baby on Malibu beach. The topic was communication in medical care!

The echo of illness and HIV was reverberating in California. Ears were pricked up and whispers of intrigue were overheard in corridors. When I returned to London and work, the National Health Service was duty-bound to honor my maternity leave, to keep me on staff until the following round of British Psychological Society examinations, another year. This placed me in the psychology department, interested in evidence-based practice, alerted to a new disease, the moment of AIDS.

So my reflections, both personal and professional, go back to the first reactions of knowledge transfer at the beginning of the epidemic, a time when change was vital and adaptation was key. Psychologists had long known that knowledge was necessary but not sufficient for behavior change. They also knew that fear arousal was not an effective intervention for behavior change. Both were clearly evidenced from the smoking and cancer campaigns. Armed with such knowledge, the governments of the day almost universally decided to respond with high-profile, fear-arousing campaigns.

The UK government was no different and hatched the idea of the iceberg adverts, with grim overtone voices warning of impending death and doom. The image warned that there was a hidden menace. The visuals included death bouquets of lilies strewn on gravestones with the caption "AIDS— don't die of ignorance"; or a floating, somber, looming, blackened iceberg with the caption "There is now a deadly virus."

These were followed by gruesome advertisements for drug users with visuals of twisted, drug-filled teaspoons melting contraband substances over clandestine flames, blood-stained syringes, and a warning against sharing needles. The slogans and messages were encapsulated with the mantra "Don't die of ignorance." Full-page advertisements with microscope images of a grainy virus were published in the national press. Advertisements appeared on national television.

In Australia, they invoked the assistance of the Grim Reaper. The Australian Department of Health published a skeleton version of the Grim Reaper, with a hatchet slung over his shoulder. The character used bowling balls to strike individuals off their feet. The campaign was withdrawn given the backlash.

My clinical thesis was based on a hurried evaluation of some of these campaigns. I gathered some pre-exposure data and then followed up groups in the sexually transmitted infections and injection drug user clinics and among medical students.

It is no surprise that we found very little effect, as the ads raised anxiety but did not provide action, and they were read with intrigue but had little impact on behavior. The targeted campaigns were not seen as relevant by the target group. The visual images of microscope views of virus were neither recognized nor understood. Medical students thought they were images of a nipple or a space rocket. The attenders at the local methadone clinic found the large scary images of drugs on teaspoons quite endearing rather than frightening, and they led to cravings rather than avoidance. Everyone thought the ads were targeted at someone else, not themselves. This probably served to feed the hype rather than solve it.

These ads heralded an avalanche of advertisements globally. Did these drive or reflect the epidemic? Did they change attitudes or behavior? Did they revolutionize knowledge levels? Did they galvanize action? On reflection, there is little sound evidence of a sea change. In fact, it may be seen as a paper panacea of the early days. In the absence of action, this was a substitute activity. Looking back at the knowledge scramble, there seem to be three phases that describe the periods from the 1980s to the present day, which can be best described as the three Ls: Leaflets, Lips, and Log on.

Leaflets refers to the abundance of quasi-information sheets, which were often written at a level not accessible by the lay reader or conversely written in such condescending tones that they insulted the informed consumer. Lengthy debates were held on how to capture all taboo subjects on single sheets of paper—sex, blood, and relationships!

Lips refers to the next phase where *dialogue* was seen as a solution pathway. This was reflected in the many support groups, the need for counseling around HIV testing (both pre-test and post-test) on the assumption that such dialogue would benefit both those with a positive HIV test result and those with a negative test result. Negotiation dialogue, support group dialogue, help lines, community engagement, and interdisciplinary dialogue all flourished. All forms typified an era of action.

The next phase was the advent and growing use of the Internet. *Log on* refers to the ability to vastly enhance reach, access knowledge, navigate systems, update evidence, gather data, or just chat. This has probably revolutionized knowledge transfer and access. Indeed the challenge now becomes knowledge management, knowledge overwhelm, knowledge navigation, and knowledge exhaustion.

Knowledge was not confined to HIV transmission knowledge. As psychologists, we also wanted to know and understand the nature of the challenges, the most effective interventions, and the counseling needs. In the absence of precedent, we approached the challenges with caution and reflection. We tried different approaches and monitored them, and we gathered psychological data and tried to understand the many facets of the epidemic, including multiple bereavement, coping and adaptation, risk reduction, managing HIV testing, burnout, side effects, and responding to opportunistic infections. In the early days, there were no care or treatment options that were viable, available, or effective. We drew on the literature of bereavement, trauma, and health psychology. Indeed, the times allowed for innovation. Some changes in healthcare practice may never have occurred if the HIV epidemic had not triggered change. This was probably the result of the confluence of a number of challenges and opportunities:

- atypical physicians drawn into the field of HIV care typified by open and patient-centered approaches
- stigmatization and discrimination as the epidemic concentrated in groups who were fighting multiple problems, which demanded a dramatic reexamination of old practices
- emergency funding that allowed for some innovation as well as evaluation
- a sense of collegiality unprecedented in other areas of academic study
- a vociferous and informed group affected by the epidemic who aspired to the view of "nothing about us without us"
- an urgency for action-based solutions rather than endless thinking and pondering
- a global challenge that required global knowledge sharing, partnerships, and action

We introduced "psychosocial ward rounds," so rather than discussing symptoms, drugs, and side effects, we discussed human reaction, support, planning, and well-being. The hierarchical models prevalent in healthcare gave way to a more multidisciplinary approach. Community action and re-action were integrated with HIV in a way that had never been seen in other health conditions.

Yet the tension between knowledge and knee-jerk persisted. On the clinical side, there was an urgency to do rather than to know. On the academic side, there was so much to be done that research questions were overwhelming.

So where did that leave me in all of this? For starters, I thought that the importance of knowledge, evidence, and clear guidance was imperative. This resulted in the launching, together in those days with Robert Bor, of the journal *AIDS Care*. The journal, under my editorship, is now produced monthly and is in its 28th year of publication. It also resulted in the launching of the AIDSImpact conference series. A group of us were disillusioned with the lack of comprehensive understanding of the psychosocial concepts and the poor handling of these issues at the international AIDS conferences.

AIDSImpact, a boutique-style conference, was set up with a band of inspirational pioneers, gathering new blood as we moved forward. The skills of Jose Catalan, Barbara Hedge, Frans van den Boom, Bruno Spire, Jean Paul Moattie, Kees Reitmeijer, Bridgette Prince, Olive Shisana, Lucie Cluver, Richard Harding, and Udi Davidovich (all ably helped by amazing local committees) ensured a dynamism embracing knowledge and disseminating it. We ran as a nonprofit and prided ourselves in our vast program of support and the number of collaborations and contributions (let alone partnerships) that emerged along our corridors.

The first meeting, spearheaded by Frans van den Boom in Amsterdam, marked the beginning of a series, stretching twice to Amsterdam, twice to the UK, as far flung as Ottowa, Melbourne, Gaberone, Marseille, Milan, Barcelona, Cape Town, and the first AIDS meeting to return to the US in Santa Fe, after lifting of travel restrictions. We were the first conference to welcome the community. Indeed, the newly created Red Ribbon campaign sent delegates to pass through the aisles during our opening ceremony and hand out red ribbons to the delegates. A precedent had been set.

The third International AIDS Society Conference in Washington, DC, marked a high-impact moment in time. The sessions were filled to overflowing, the talks were broadcast on national television, and people grasped for knowledge. I have attended all subsequent IAS conferences and watched the political and care agendas roller coaster through time.

In my clinical department at St. Mary's, research was seen as secondary to the demands of clinical care. I took one day a week unpaid to continue research and then realized that the pursuit of knowledge, the dissemination of findings, and the evidence-based interventions were actually a form of clinical care, simply operating at a higher level.

In 1993, I left St. Mary's and went to the warm enfolding arms of a university environment, the University College London. I have remained there ever since as a long-term survivor in the knowledge race.

Methadone Treatment, Jessie Helms, and Reaching Women Who Use Drugs

WENDEE M. WECHSBERG

I MOVED TO North Carolina in 1984 to run an outpatient drug treatment program. Soon after, North Carolina's State Health Director, Ron Levine, created a task force to address AIDS. Locally, we also started a task force to establish the AIDS Service Agency, now called the AIDS Alliance, which over the years has grown to cover the state. I was the local methadone treatment director and represented the injecting drug user community. Methadone treatment was still getting mixed reviews as an opioid replacement therapy. Addicts have long faced stigmatization, as have addicts on methadone treatment. Over the years through education and with famous people sharing their stories, the addiction field has achieved greater compassion. However, more than 30 years ago when we mostly had methadone programs and persons newly infected with HIV, there was a lack of knowledge about HIV and essentially no treatment protocols like we have today. Mostly what we had was our understanding that we were dealing with something big and unknown and our commitment to dealing with it. This was an important juncture that dramatically changed my career path.

We thought we were being revolutionary to begin HIV counseling and testing in the methadone program in Raleigh as soon as the test was available. At the time, we believed that people had very little time to live once they had full-blown AIDS. We used to say two years, then we said five years. It was also a time when Senator Jesse Helms had achieved significant notoriety, and he lived not too far from our clinic.

I will never forget our first HIV-positive test result with a larger-than-life, African American male patient. It did not go well. He was very angry. He threatened the staff, so I had to intervene and eventually escort him out of the clinic, but not before he asserted that he was going to "f—k every young thing he knows to spread this disease." I was shaken, but it made me realize that we needed to do more. At the time, North Carolina only had isolation and quarantine laws on the public health books for a situation like this where others might be in danger. We felt helpless. However, it was that salient moment that was the turning point in my career.

I decided to develop an education program for our injecting drug users and take it on the road to the other treatment programs in the state to promote risk reduction. We applied for a Centers for Disease Control grant through the state to start outreach in public housing communities and distribute methadone clinic coupons to injecting drug users to increase entry into methadone treatment. The grant was approved for funding; however, I was required to remove the bleach and water risk-reduction kits. These kits were for injecting drug users who were not ready for treatment, to reduce their risk of being infected with the virus. But because of a special Helms amendment, the kits could not be funded. No government funds could be perceived as "enabling" the drug problem.

It was frustrating. Nonetheless, we established outreach with recovering addicts and our methadone program grew. Sadly, the first outreach worker in the field relapsed, which taught us to make sure that outreach workers work in teams and have at least two years of sobriety.

During that time, I also wrote a small grant to the Robert Wood Johnson Foundation, and it was awarded to us as well. The Foundation did not care that we wanted to offer bleach and water kits, and with added support, this allowed us to expand to several low-income communities where ongoing drug use was known to persist. We reached thousands through our educational outreach efforts, and our census in the methadone program doubled at that point from the treatment coupons.[1]

The publicity surrounding the Helms amendment and these risk-reduction efforts made the local press. Of course, the activism was unabashed. It was strong, and we all became very close, feeling we were in the fight together for something important. The state and local efforts were developing at the same time.

Scott Hustead and Nat Blevins became two of my friends as we developed a statewide AIDS strategy. Then the unimaginable happened—Scott was hospitalized with *Pneumocystis carinii* pneumonia. We talked by phone, because I didn't have a babysitter for my young children so that I could go see him in the hospital in Chapel Hill. He sounded so weak, but said, "Don't worry, I am getting out tomorrow." However, he died the next day. It was quite a personal shock that he was gone just like that and made me realize we weren't moving fast enough. Scott's memorial was at Duke Gardens and was filled with so much love.

We planned to open our first AIDS care house under Scott's name, but it turned out not to be so easy. There were "not in my neighborhood!" demonstrations in Raleigh, with neighbors hating the idea of the Hustead House. I clearly remember the walk, starting at the local church, and the signs. Ironically, those neighbors ended up being great supporters and volunteers. Isn't it interesting how time creates understanding and healing? Before he died, even Jesse Helms apologized about some of his misunderstandings about HIV and AIDS. I wished I had talked with him before he died.

Nat Blevins went on to work in Washington at the President's Commission on AIDS. I remember him picking me up to give some testimony on injection drug use. He was also very sick, covering himself in the car with a colorful Mexican blanket to keep warm. The care house in Durham was then named the Blevins House. It's so very sad that my two good friends in the fight left so soon.

Then someone said to me, if I wanted to do this in a greater fashion, I needed my PhD. So even as a single parent, I gave up being a methadone director in 1989 to get a PhD in community psychology so I could expand this work through research and practice. I said I would never give up working in addiction, having once been an addict and losing my father to addiction. My commitment to the addiction field remains unwavering to this day.

My intervention work in HIV expanded from North Carolina to South Africa and other regions of the world where HIV is a scourge, especially for women, who carry the greater burden of this disease globally. Gender inequalities and the nexus of substance use, gender-based violence, and sexual risk have kept me focused on HIV for three decades. I was lucky when I got my first National Institutes of Health AIDS grant the year after I got out of graduate school and then another . . . and I have been gratefully funded to do HIV-related interventions ever since, knowing that focus, passion, and persistence pay off.

My first projects were funded by the National Institute on Drug Abuse (NIDA) in 1994 and 1995. Over the years they have evolved into multiple adaptations of a woman-focused HIV prevention intervention. It was obvious that we needed to do something different for women who use drugs. We formed a workgroup at NIDA to develop interventions to reach women, some of whom were injecting drug users and some not. In the 1990s we had a crack cocaine epidemic in North Carolina, and HIV was increasing among African American women. (In the South the majority of HIV cases were among African American women, and that has not changed to this day.) Many of these women who used crack found themselves trading sex to maintain their addiction, and they were involved in other risky behaviors, including unprotected sex or inconsistent condom use, longer crack runs, increased number of sex partners, violence, homelessness, and alcohol use.[2,3] They also reported separation from their children.[4] These complexities were the impetus for an empowering woman-focused intervention called the Women's CoOp, which was developed to reduce homelessness, increase employment, and reduce risky behaviors.[5]

The original Women's CoOp was considered a best-evidence intervention by the CDC[6] and was adapted in North Carolina for pregnant African American women who used drugs[7] and for African American teens who had dropped out of school or were at risk of dropping out of school, were sexually active, and used drugs.[8] There was also a follow-on study four to seven years later to determine what happened to the women who used crack. Almost 10 percent of these women were living with HIV. However, long-term, these findings were mixed with the issues surrounding addiction and recovery. Some women were doing better, some the same, some were worse; and over time, some with no intervention were doing better, akin to a sleeper effect.[9] The bottom line about addiction and risk of HIV is that we need to keep at it with innovative interventions because incidence continues with African American women in the South.

North Carolina was also doing a good job of reaching these HIV-positive women with housing and medication, with the success of the Center for AIDS Research at the University of North Carolina at Chapel Hill and Duke University School of Medicine. In fact, in one focus group discussion, a woman said that it's almost better to be a "a positive woman in this community" because she felt these women got housing over other women.

About the same time, South Africa was reporting that one in four women in their antenatal programs were HIV positive, and after a talk on the North Carolina Women's CoOp at NIDA, the head of NIDA's Medical Consequences Office requested that I consider expanding to South Africa in 2001. At first it was daunting, but after the initial pilot, several other studies followed with women who used drugs, many of whom were sex workers living with HIV. We found high rates of HIV, especially among sex workers, which has persisted in South Africa with women who use alcohol and other drugs, as shown in numerous studies funded by NIDA, the National Institute on Alcohol Abuse and Alcoholism, and the Eunice Kennedy Shriver National Institute of Child Health and Human Development.[10]

We worked on several adaptations of the intervention to address the gender-based violence we found that women were experiencing in South Africa. We also realized if we wanted to help women, we needed to reach men. So we took two years to develop a men's intervention and to adapt another one for couples.[11] In all of the studies, we targeted very poor, vulnerable, and key populations because of their substance use and condomless sex. We also incorporated the dimension of gender roles, communication, and sexy safe sex to promote monogymy. We found serodiscordance among couples, with women two times more likely to be infected with HIV than men.[12]

But we can't just keep adapting interventions and testing how well they work. We also need to move to the next phase. Recently, we've started marketing the Women's Health CoOp within an implementation science framework for adoption and sustainability in both health departments and drug treatment programs in South Africa for women living with HIV. The importance of addressing alcohol and drug use, sexuality, and violence prevention along with teaching healthy behaviors may increase adherence as well as improve structural factors within these settings.

Who knows what will be in the next 30 years, bearing in mind the UNAIDS 90-90-90 target (that 90 percent of people with HIV will know their status, 90 percent of those will be receiving treatment, and 90 percent of those will be virally suppressed)? However, high HIV incidence continues in the communities in which we work, and adherence to HIV medication is a challenge because of ongoing alcohol and drug use. We also know that we need to reach more men, because they are transmitting HIV to women, and many are not getting tested.

Looking back and looking forward, we know that we are not done. Many careers have developed with these projects, many friendships have been forged, many staff have become family, and our own children have grown up. When I look back at the moments that drive my passion to do this work, I remember that first threatening patient and how Jesse Helms kept us from using bleach and water. Yet today we are able to give out new needles. There has been great progress.

Yet, I remember Scott and Nat. I remember the activism. Today I worry about apathy. We know so much more about HIV—how to prevent it and how to care for it as a chronic disease. Maybe a cure is even close at hand. But in South Africa, people are hungry, so taking medication is secondary to survival. They like to drink, so they take "holidays" from taking ARV medications. Stigma is still rampant and healthcare staff are stressed and often burned out. My generation is losing the first generation of people committed to preventing and ending HIV, and we hope that through mentoring, the next generation will take up the torch. We need inspired, willing, passionate people who know that the work isn't easy but that every life is worth it.

As a post note, there is a new crisis with opiate addiction and sadly with it, too many overdose deaths. In every paper there is a story, and it is getting congressional attention. New dollars are being made available for treatment, and ironically, because of this turn of events, last year the governor of North Carolina approved needle exchange. Some things take a long time. This new crisis will bring new injecting behavior and likely new spread of disease, whether it be hepatitis C or HIV. As said, there is always much to be done.

Acknowledgments

In gratitude for funding under NIDA R03 DA009001; NIDA U01 DA008007; NIDA R01 DA011609; NIDA R01 DA011609-S1; NIDA R01 DA020852; CDC UR6 PS000665; NIAAA R01 AA014488; NICHD R01 HD058320; NIAAA R01 AA018076; and NIAAA R01 AA022882.

References

1. Wechsberg WM, Smith FJ, Harris-Adeeyo T. AIDS education and outreach to IV drug users and the community: strategies and results. Psychol Addict Behav. 1992;6(2):107–13.

2. Edwards JM, Halpern CT, Wechsberg WM. Correlates of exchanging sex for drugs or money among women who use crack cocaine. AIDS Educ Prev 2006;18(5):420–9.

3. Wechsberg WM, Lam WK, Zule W, Hall G, Middlesteadt R, Edwards J. Violence, homelessness, and HIV risk among crack-using African-American women. Subst Use Misuse 2003;38(3–6):669–700.

4. Lam WK, Wechsberg W, Zule W. African-American women who use crack cocaine: a comparison of mothers who live with and have been separated from their children. Child Abuse Negl 2004;28(11):1229–47.

5. Wechsberg WM, Lam WK, Zule WA, Bobashev G. Efficacy of a woman-focused intervention to reduce HIV risk and increase self-sufficiency among African American crack abusers. Am J Public Health 2004;94(7):1165–73.

6. Lyles CM, Kay LS, Crepaz N, Herbst JH, Passin WF, Kim AS, et al. Best-evidence interventions: findings from a systematic review of HIV behavioral interventions for US populations at high risk, 2000–2004. Am J Public Health 2007;97(1):133–43.

7. Wechsberg WM, Browne FA, Poulton W, Ellerson RM, Simons-Rudolph A, Haller D. Adapting an evidence-based HIV prevention intervention for

pregnant African-American women in substance abuse treatment. Subst Abuse Rehabil 2011;2(1):35–42.

8. Wechsberg WM, Browne FA, Zule WA, Novak SP, Doherty IA, Kline TL, et al. Efficacy of the Young Women's CoOp: an HIV risk-reduction intervention for substance-using African-American female adolescents in the South. J Child Adolesc Subst Abuse. 2017;26(3):205–18.

9. Wechsberg WM, Novak SP, Zule WA, Browne FA, Kral AH, Ellerson RM, et al. Sustainability of intervention effects of an evidence-based HIV prevention intervention for African American women who smoke crack cocaine. Drug Alcohol Depend 2010;109(1–3):205–12.

10. Wechsberg WM, Browne FA, Ellerson RM, Zule WA. Adapting the evidence-based Women's CoOp intervention to prevent human immunodeficiency virus infection in North Carolina and international settings. N C Med J 2010;71(5):477–81.

11. Wechsberg WM, El-Bassel N, Carney T, Browne FA, Myers B, Zule WA. Adapting an evidence-based HIV behavioral intervention for South African couples. Subst Abuse Treat Prev Policy 2015;10:6.

12. Wechsberg WM, Zule WA, El-Bassel N, Doherty IA, Minnis AM, Novak SD, et al. The male factor: outcomes from a cluster randomized field experiment with a couples-based HIV prevention intervention in a South African township. Drug Alcohol Depend 2016;161:307–15.

South Africa's Response to AIDS and Preventing HIV in Young Women

QUARRAISHA ABDOOL KARIM AND SALIM S. ABDOOL KARIM

OUR JOURNEY IN THE FIELD of HIV began over 30 years ago. Quar-raisha embarked on her graduate studies with a bachelor's degree from the University of Durban-Westville, majoring in microbiology and biochemistry in 1981. In 1983, she completed an Honours degree at the University of the Witwatersrand in medical biochemistry with a special focus on autoimmune diseases and genetics. During these studies, she worked with Dr. Ruben Sher, who at the time was describing and treating some of the first cases of AIDS in South Africa. Intrigued by this new disease, she decided to pursue her interest in blood-borne diseases by joining the Department of Hematology at the Faculty of Medicine of the University of Witwatersrand before joining the Department of Hematology at the Faculty of Medicine of the University of Natal in 1985.

Salim had graduated with a medical degree in 1984 from the University of Natal in Durban and completed his internship at King Edward VIII Hospital in Durban. His research interest at the time was hepatitis B, and he embarked on specialist training in the Department of Virology at the University of Natal in 1986, where he lectured medical students about HIV and worked with Isobel Windsor in providing HIV test results to patients.

Our paths crossed in 1986 when we were based in different departments at the University of Natal and we both decided in 1987 to study public health and epidemiology at the School of Public Health at Columbia University in New York. While at Columbia, we were inundated with talks on HIV. One of the really exciting talks that we recall was a public lecture by Dr. Sam Broder who spoke about his AZT trial, the first antiretroviral (ARV) drug to treat HIV. We also benefited immensely from the mentorship of Drs. Zena Stein and Mervyn Susser, who were both active in AIDS research at the time and encouraged us to conduct epidemiological studies on HIV in South Africa.

Upon our return to South Africa from Columbia University in 1989, Salim went on to complete his fellowship in Community Health at the University of Natal and Quarraisha joined the South African Medical Research Council (MRC) in Durban, where she founded the MRC AIDS Research Programme and shortly thereafter started her research on HIV and South African women.

We conducted our first joint HIV study, one of the first household surveys of HIV in South Africa, in 1989. Initially, we focused on understanding the obstacles to the uptake of HIV prevention options. The study, which was conducted in Lamontville (a peri-urban township in the south of Durban), explored the sexual behavior and knowledge of AIDS among Black mothers of teenagers and their role in communicating HIV risk to their children. The study revealed that marriage was rare, but mothers had serial monogamous relationships resulting in children from different partners; that condom use was rare; and that communication with teenage children about HIV and contraception was nonexistent.[1]

In 1990, we undertook the first population-based HIV survey, which piggybacked on the active Malaria Surveillance Program, in KwaZulu-Natal.[2] This survey highlighted that while South Africa was at an early stage of the epidemic, HIV was spreading rapidly and was disproportionately affecting young women and teenage girls, as well as adult men (Figure 11.1). This age-sex difference in HIV acquisition set us on the path to identify the biological and behavioral reasons for women's vulnerability to HIV and served as the basis of our research on HIV prevention methods for women.

In 1993, Salim joined the MRC and was appointed as director of the MRC's Centre for Epidemiological Research in South Africa (CERSA). Our research at the MRC focused on HIV, hepatitis B, and immunization. We launched our research on the development of new safe and effective HIV prevention technologies for women. Our early research in this area made important contributions to the newly emerging field of vaginal microbicides—chemical products that women can apply in the vagina to prevent HIV and other sexually transmitted infections (STIs)—and in 1993 we developed and undertook one of the earliest studies on vaginal microbicides. This study investigated the effects of nonoxynol-9 film on the vaginal epithelium and viral shedding.[3] We subsequently participated in conducting the large multicenter efficacy trial on COL-1492, a long-duration nonoxynol-9 gel.[4] Unfortunately, nonxynol-9 in both film and gel form did not

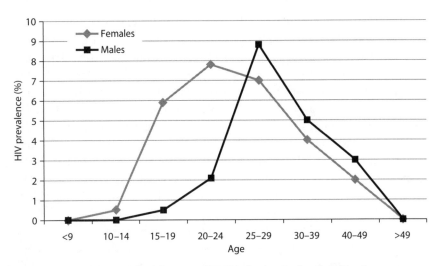

FIGURE 11.1. Age-sex distribution of HIV infection in South Africa in 1992.

protect women from HIV; in fact, this surfactant may have actually increased the risk of HIV.

Following the negative findings from the COL-1492 trial, research on surfactants came to an end. However, investigation started on a new class of candidate microbicides, polyanion gels. Salim led the team that conducted the phase I trial of PRO 2000,[5] which demonstrated that this polyanion microbicide was safe across a range of doses. He then led, as principal investigator and protocol chair, the HPTN 035 trial that assessed the safety and effectiveness of PRO 2000 gel in a $90 million six-country phase II/IIb trial funded by the US National Institutes of Health (NIH). While the overall results[6] were disappointing, an adherence analysis suggested some promise in preventing HIV. In a separate trial, this microbicide gel was found to have no impact on a woman's risk of becoming infected with HIV.

In 1994, Quarraisha was appointed by the newly established Mandela government to create the National HIV/AIDS and Sexually Transmitted Infection Programme in the Ministry of Health and we moved to Pretoria. During this time, in addition to gaining substantial policy and programming experience, she served as special advisor to the minister of health, who was also the chair of the UNAIDS (Joint United Nations Programme on HIV/AIDS) Advisory Board. She was appointed as a member of the International AIDS Society (IAS) Governing Council, and in 1996 she and Gustaaf Wolvaardt, a South African health attaché based in Geneva, submitted a bid to host the 13th International AIDS Conference in Durban in 2000.

South Africa's Response to AIDS and Preventing HIV in Women   79

The decision to host the 13th International AIDS Conference in Durban was announced in 1998, with Hoosen (Jerry) Coovadia as the conference chair and Salim as the scientific program chair. Ironically, as preparations for the conference got under way, the president of South Africa, Thabo Mbeki, started to express his views that HIV is not the cause of AIDS and that AIDS was a racist concept, with Blacks being labeled as sexual predators and promiscuous people. He used Internet-trolled information from AIDS dissidents to conclude that "a virus cannot cause a syndrome"—and by implication, that HIV cannot cause AIDS. He even established an AIDS panel on the eve of the conference composed of leading AIDS scientists—including the co-discoverer of HIV, Françoise Barré-Sinoussi—and AIDS dissidents to debate this issue.

While hundreds of South African adults and children were dying of AIDS, Mbeki's dissident position catalyzed the creation of a civil society movement, the Treatment Action Campaign. The Treatment Action Campaign rallied grassroots support and unity in the local response to the epidemic as well as global support and solidarity, resulting in the release of the Durban Declaration, which laid out unequivocally the scientific basis of HIV as the cause of AIDS. In contrast, it was particularly striking to note how Mbeki's cabinet, parliament, and more broadly the African National Congress defended Mbeki, seeing an attack on him as an attack on the African National Congress. The country had not been so divided since the transition to democracy. It took the presence and words of former president Nelson Mandela at the closing of the 13th International AIDS Conference to convene a special cabinet meeting that weekend, where a commitment was made to provide antiretroviral treatment to AIDS patients.

While the conference was a resounding success and was recognized as a turning point in the HIV epidemic by serving as a catalyst to end the injustice of global inequity in access to AIDS treatment, Mbeki's minister of health, Tshabalala-Msimang, remained his defender-in-chief and saw to it that ARVs were not provided by the state. She was aided by several provincial members of the executive council (MECs), including MEC Manase in Mpumalanga and MEC Nkonyeni in KwaZulu-Natal. The provision of ARV treatment through PEPFAR and the Global Fund for AIDS, Tuberculosis and Malaria, in partnership with nongovernmental organizations and academic institutions, enabled hundreds of thousands of lives to be saved. The change in administration in 2007 with President Kgalema Montlanthe and Minister of Health Barbara Hogan initiated a more fitting response to the HIV epidemic that has grown in Jacob Zuma's administration with

Dr. Aron Motsoaledi, as minister of health, serving as the key driver of the HIV response.

In 1997, Salim led the team that applied to the Wellcome Trust to create a new £5 million HIV research center in rural KwaZulu-Natal. With a successful bid to establish the Africa Centre for Population Studies and Reproductive Health, we relocated back to Durban and Salim took up the position of director at the Africa Centre, where the research focused on sexually transmitted infections and understanding the drivers of the HIV epidemic in KwaZulu-Natal.

In 1998, Quarraisha rejoined the MRC as a senior epidemiologist in the AIDS Programme of CERSA. Here she gained experience in undertaking intervention research, including clinical trials, through several successful NIH grants. In parallel, she coordinated the Columbia University–Southern African Fogarty AIDS Training Programme. This program was key to building the science base in South Africa to enhance the responses to the AIDS and TB epidemics by training over 600 basic scientists, clinician researchers, and epidemiologists. Quarraisha completed her PhD in 2000 on the epidemiology of HIV infection in women in South Africa at the University of Natal, under the mentorship of Professors Jerry Coovadia and Jack Moodley. Shortly thereafter, she was appointed as assistant professor at Columbia University and moved to the University of Natal. Salim also moved to the University of Natal, as deputy vice-chancellor for research.

In 2001, the NIH's Comprehensive International Program of Research on AIDS (CIPRA) funding announcement presented a unique opportunity for South African scientists, in collaboration with leading US scientists, to make a new and significant contribution to AIDS research. We at the University of Natal—together with a team of senior scientists from South Africa from the University of Cape Town, University of Western Cape, and the National Institute of Communicable Diseases and from Columbia University—decided to combine our efforts to establish a multidisciplinary collaborative program known as the Centre for the AIDS Programme of Research in South Africa (CAPRISA).

With the creation of CAPRISA we were able to gain a better understanding of the gender differences in HIV prevalence and the age-related behavioral and biological factors driving the epidemic. In addition to our research on HIV and TB co-treatment and our studies on acute HIV infection, we also focused on young rural women, who have among the highest HIV incidence rates observed globally.

Following a decade of disappointments in developing a safe and effective woman-controlled HIV prevention option, we decided in 2004 to pursue a novel approach based on interesting new data from studies in monkeys. This approach involved testing an AIDS treatment medication as a microbicidal gel to prevent HIV. Using the ARV drug tenofovir, acquired from Gilead Sciences, we proceeded in 2007 to conduct clinical studies of this drug in a vaginally applied gel formulation. We co-led the CAPRISA 004 trial that went on to prove the concept[7] that ARVs can prevent sexually acquired HIV infection in women and subsequently that high tenofovir levels were essential[8] to achieve high levels of protection. This landmark finding has been heralded by UNAIDS and the World Health Organization as one of the most significant scientific breakthroughs in the fight against AIDS and was ranked by *Science* as one of the top 10 scientific breakthroughs of 2010. This study also showed that tenofovir gel prevents genital herpes (HSV-2),[9] an incurable lifelong condition, which potentiates the spread of HIV infection.

While exciting, these results alone were not sufficient to license tenofovir gel for HIV prevention. There was high hope that the ongoing Microbicide Trials Network's VOICE (Vaginal and Oral Interventions to Control the Epidemic) trial,[10] which included daily use of tenofovir gel, would confirm the results from the CAPRISA 004 trial. Disappointingly, none of the three products—tenofovir gel, oral tenofovir disoproxil fumarate (TDF), or oral coformulated emtricitabine and tenofovir (Truvada)—tested in the VOICE trial were shown to be effective in preventing HIV.[10] An analysis of detectable drug levels in blood showed that few of the VOICE participants adhered to the daily dosing regimen: adherence was estimated to be 23 percent, 28 percent, and 29 percent with the tenofovir gel, oral tenofovir, and oral Truvada, respectively.[10] The Follow-on African Consortium for Tenofovir Studies 001 (FACTS 001), which was designed as a confirmatory study for the CAPRISA 004 trial, also produced disappointing results, showing that tenofovir gel had no impact on HIV.[11] In the FACTS 001 trial about half of the women in the trial had detectable drug levels.[11] Both of these studies highlight the importance of achieving high adherence in microbicide trials.

Our HIV research on tenofovir gel has continued, and our subsequent key findings on tenofovir concentrations as a potential surrogate marker of protection,[8] the role of genital inflammation in enhancing HIV acquisition,[12] the role of impaired innate immune responses in increasing HIV susceptibility,[13] and the role of the vaginal microbiome[14] are already having an impact on the design and testing of next-generation microbicides. Our research has also contributed to addressing some of the methodological challenges associated with microbicide trials[15] regarding novel adherence strategies and measurement,[16,17] which are now being used in several other microbicide trials.

Our HIV prevention research has now shifted toward provision of pre-exposure prophylaxis (PrEP) to young women to inform policy and practice and the developmental research on long-acting ARV products that potentially decrease adherence challenges. Our ongoing epidemiological studies[18] continue to provide a nuanced understanding of the evolving and dynamic nature of the HIV epidemic and shape the development of HIV prevention and treatment efforts and surveillance efforts.[19] These studies continue to inform our research priorities, policy and programmatic-level priorities,[20] which have a focus on HIV prevention in adolescent women as a key driver to the epidemic in southern Africa and are critical to altering epidemic trajectories in the region.[21] TB-HIV coinfection continues to be a key reason we continue to see people dying from AIDS, despite having one of the largest treatment programs. Stigma and discrimination continue to be a major barrier to knowledge of HIV status.

While we have made immense progress and substantial contributions to understanding the evolving HIV epidemic, providing a more granular understanding of HIV risk in young women and advancing women-initiated prevention technologies, this journey is far from over. It has and continues to be a special privilege to work with scientists, activists, communities, sponsors, and research participants across South Africa and globally with the unity of purpose to end AIDS.

References

1. Abdool Karim Q, Abdool Karim SS, Nkomokazi J. Sexual behaviour and knowledge of AIDS among urban black mothers. Implications for AIDS intervention programmes. S Afr Med J 1991;80(7):340–3.

2. Abdool Karim Q, Abdool Karim SS, Singh B, Short R, Ngxongo S. Seroprevalence of HIV infection in rural South Africa. AIDS 1992;6(12):1535–9.

3. Rustomjee R, Abdool Karim Q, Abdool Karim SS, Laga M, Stein Z. Phase 1 trial of nonoxynol-9 film among sex workers in South Africa. AIDS 1999;13(12):1511–5.

4. Van Damme L, Ramjee G, Alary M, Vuylsteke B, Chandeying V, Rees H, et al. Effectiveness of COL-1492, a nonoxynol-9 vaginal gel, on HIV-1 transmission in female sex workers: a randomised controlled trial. Lancet 2002;360(9338): 971–7.

5. Mayer KH, Karim SA, Kelly C, Maslankowski L, Rees H, Profy AT, et al. Safety and tolerability of vaginal PRO 2000 gel in sexually active HIV-uninfected and abstinent HIV-infected women. AIDS 2003;17(3):321–9.

6. Abdool Karim SS, Richardson B, Ramjee G, Hoffman I, Chirenje M, Taha T, et al. Safety and effectiveness of BufferGel and 0.5% PRO2000 gel for the prevention of HIV infection in women. AIDS 2010;25:957–66.

7. Abdool Karim Q, Abdool Karim SS, Frohlich JA, Grobler AC, Baxter C, Mansoor LE, et al. Effectiveness and safety of tenofovir gel, an antiretroviral microbicide, for the prevention of HIV infection in women. Science 2010; 329(5996):1168–74.

8. Abdool Karim SS, Kashuba A, Werner L, Abdool Karim Q. Drug concentrations following topical and oral antiretroviral pre-exposure prophylaxis: implications for HIV prevention in women. Lancet 2011;378:279–81.

9. Abdool Karim SS, Abdool Karim Q, Kharsany AB, Baxter C, Grobler AC, Werner L, et al. Tenofovir gel for the prevention of herpes simplex virus type 2 infection. N Engl J Med 2015;373(6):530–9.

10. Marrazzo JM, Ramjee G, Richardson BA, Gomez K, Mgodi N, Nair G, et al. Tenofovir-based preexposure prophylaxis for HIV infection among African women. N Engl J Med 2015;372(6):509–18.

11. Rees H, Delany-Moretlwe S.A., Lombard C, Baron D, Panchia R, Myer L, et al. Facts 001 phase III trial of pericoital tenofovir 1% gel for HIV prevention in women. [abstract 26lb]. Conference on Retroviruses and Opportunistic Infections (CROI); Seattle, WA; 23–26 Feb 2015.

12. Masson L, Passmore JA, Liebenberg LJ, Werner L, Baxter C, Arnold KB, et al. Genital inflammation and the risk of HIV acquisition in women. Clin Infect Dis 2015;61(2):260–9.

13. Naranbhai V, Abdool Karim SS, Altfeld M, Samsunder N, Durgiah R, Sibeko S, et al. Innate immune activation enhances HIV acquisition in women, diminishing the effectiveness of tenofovir microbicide gel. J Infect Dis 2012; 206(7):993–1001.

14. Abdool Karim SS, editor. Understanding high rates of HIV in young women in Africa: implications of new epidemiological, phylogenetic, genomic and proteomic evidence. In: AIDS 2016; Durban, South Africa; 2016.

15. Grobler AC, Abdool Karim SS. Design challenges facing clinical trials of the effectiveness of new HIV-prevention technologies. AIDS 2012;26(5):529–32.

16. Mansoor LE, Abdool Karim Q, Yende-Zuma N, MacQueen KM, Baxter C, Madlala B, et al. Adherence in the CAPRISA 004 tenofovir gel microbicide trial. AIDS Behav 2014;18(5):811–9.

17. Gengiah TN, Mansoor LE, Upfold M, Naidoo A, Yende-Zuma N, Kashuba AD, et al. Measuring adherence by visual inspection of returned empty gel applicators in the CAPRISA 004 microbicide trial. AIDS Behav 2014;18(5): 820–5.

18. Abdool Karim Q, Kharsany AB, Frohlich JA, Werner L, Mashego M, Mlotshwa M, et al. Stabilizing HIV prevalence masks high HIV incidence rates amongst rural and urban women in KwaZulu-Natal, South Africa. Int J Epidemiol. 2011;40(4):922–30.

19. Abdool Karim S, Abdool Karim Q. The evolving HIV epidemic in South Africa. Int J of Epidemiology. 2002;31:37–40.

20. Abdool Karim SS, Abdool Karim Q. AIDS research must link to local policy. Nature. 2010;463(7282):733–4.

21. Abdool Karim Q, Sibeko S, Baxter C. Preventing HIV infection in women: a global health imperative. Clin Infect Dis. 2010;50 Suppl 3:S122–9.

Survivors

Finding the Black Church in the Fight to End AIDS

My Story

BISHOP STACEY S. LATIMER

I WAS BORN AND RAISED in the Bible Belt, in South Carolina. If there is one thing that I remember about my childhood it is my love for my local house of worship. I was the baby of the family, not yet six years old, waking up the entire house to make sure we were not going to be late for worship service. I remember at the age of five, I was drawn by the music and what it stirred in my spirit. The gift that music gave to the service was almost magical, definitely mystical. There was no other place like "church" for me.

I wasn't quite five years old when I discovered the Lord had gifted me musically to play the piano. Every Sunday after service I would sneak to the back of the building into the Sunday school area and fiddle around on the piano, while no one else was around. One Sunday, by surprise, the organist returned to the area and unbeknownst to me, she stood and listened. "When did you learn how to play?" she asked. "I'm just messing around," I replied. "You are playing what I played in service earlier," she said. "Really?" I asked.

Ironically, about seven months later my oldest sister asked my parents for permission to take piano lessons. They agreed, and in less than two weeks we arrived home from school to a piano sitting in the living room. Everyone in the house was excited. My sister immediately began her piano lessons. It was three days later, on an early Saturday morning that I sat down and began to play. The sound of music made its way down the hallways, under the doors, into rooms, and fell on the ears of those awake and sleeping. My mother, who was in the bathroom, came running to the living room doorway. She stood there, staring in amazement with a proud smile on her face. Before I knew it my three sisters were all standing in the doorway as well, looking very surprised.

Late that evening when my dad returned from a business trip, I was playing piano, unaware of his arrival. After I made eye contact with him, he continued to stand there a few more seconds then walked away without saying a word. The next couple of days there was this awkwardness in the house. Then on Thursday of the following week, my sisters and I returned from school, exited the school bus, and began walking up the driveway. We met my dad in his truck coming down the driveway with the piano secured on the back. Immediately I begin to scream and cry uncontrollably. "Where are you taking my piano?" Over and over I pleaded for an answer. Finally my dad responded with the answer that broke my heart. He said to me, "Men don't play pianos."

The part missing from this real-life account that brings more understanding is that as a child I was very feminine. The name given to my ways in the 1960s and 1970s was "sissy." It was evident that my dad loved me. But in reality he had not been prepared by anyone to raise a gay son. The culture, custom, and religion labeled homosexuality as an abomination to God, a mental disorder; therefore to the people who believed in God, they were to believe the same. Many Believers hold to that standard today. Nevertheless, there was no one-two-three step manual for him to read or training for him to attend. He only had what had been given him by his father, guidance from the pulpit, cultural norms and traditions, and the love for me that he held in his heart.

As a people, our history reflects that Black people born in America were born into a system of oppression of the worst kind. As a people, we have witnessed and experienced hate in ways beyond the mistreatment of animals. A people stripped of their identity, dignity, religion, and land. Even in the 21st century we are still healing, recovering, and overcoming. We are still flittering through, processing this maze filled with ideologies, theories, and predictions that place Black people at the bottom of the bottom.

The Black Church, for Black people, has been and remains the vessel of righteousness that affords Black people the Savior, in Jesus Christ. In Christ we are blessed, as our forefathers were able to acquire the strength to forgive and overcome the impossible. This power came from their God, the forgiver of their sins. A heart open to agape—the highest form of love and charity, the love of God for humankind and humankind's love for God—is open to the miraculous strength of the God that created all things. The Black Church has been and is the cornerstone for Black life, Black living, and Black survival.

The Specter of HIV

HIV has not only had an impact on the physical lives of individuals; it also exposed and challenged the love ethic of families, houses of worship, and the traditional norms communities place on relationships, sex, and sexuality. Despite advances in HIV/AIDS prevention and treatment, the enormous human suffering caused in terms of death, disability, loss of livelihood, and discrimination reached pandemic proportions before the Black community, including the Black Church, was officially notified. As the epidemic now moves past year 35, data continue to show that the brunt of the pandemic, along with a growing surge, is in Black communities.

History holds an account of great activism pertaining to justice and care on the part of the Black Church. Since its inception, the Black Church has rallied and stood on the front lines and in the trenches and in the courtroom for every issue pertaining to its constituents' health, life, and freedom. It has advocated tirelessly when anything threatened the safety of its members. Yet key questions remain unanswered. Where is the Black Church in advocating for the care of their constituents who have been infected with and affected by HIV/AIDS? Where is the Black Church in the fight to end AIDS in Black communities?

Caught Off Guard

The media depicted HIV/AIDS as a disease prevalent among gay white males. But while researchers were focusing on this segment of the population, African Americans were also being infected. Hospitals were seeing increasing numbers of African American patients with rare forms of pneumonia, lymphoma, and infections now commonly known to be symptomatic of HIV infection. Seemingly few, if any, physicians made the connection between these African Americans and this "gay" disease. As she tried to grasp the depth of what was happening through lenses obstructed by a religious culture and tradition saturated in sexism and ingrained with homophobia, the Black Church found herself caught off guard, gripped by fear, and paralyzed by a theology unprepared to grapple with the scourge of AIDS.

Because typically people knew so little about sexuality and the culture of the times, and particularly about "Black culture," and rejected same-sex love as unnatural, the association between gay males and AIDS brought up images in people's minds of promiscuous behavior and a sexuality that many African American males, especially religious leaders, vehemently condemned. African American males, in general, despite the private preferences of some, publicly reject homosexuality. Among this population of men whose manhood has been and continues to be under attack, homophobia breeds contempt that often manifests itself in fire-and-brimstone sermons laced with moral judgment and condemnation. Many male African American religious leaders, even today, regard AIDS as punishment, a deserved damnation. Consequently, it is not surprising that many of the first HIV prevention programs started in African American communities, including faith communities, were started by women. Such vehement rejection by the Black Church, the apex of the African American community, instilled fear of personal rejection by everyone. This fear pushed the issue of HIV/AIDS and all it encompasses underground. Families remained silent while watching loved ones suffer and die.

Another 10 years would pass, even though there were outcries from Black leaders—such as the late Dr. Beny Primm and Congresswoman Maxine Waters and others—before the public was informed that this bloodborne disease had never been restricted to the gay community. By the time the medical industry acknowledged these facts, over 60 percent of all new infections were occurring among African American men, women, and children, who collectively comprise less than 13 percent of the US population.

My Internal War

Toward the end of my junior year at university, the fight between the truth of my sexuality and theology caused me great trepidation. The internal war was hidden from most, but my dysfunctional behavior over a period of time compounded my dysfunction, which ended with me taking every pill I had in the medicine cabinet. Allergy and sinus issues—the cabinet was well stocked. The doctor recommended that I take a year off from school and get therapy. Therapists, counselors, psychiatrists, and psychologists were associated with mental health. In Black communities, needing to see one of these professionals was a sign that someone was "crazy."

I joined the Armed Forces in 1985, thinking that was the best thing for me to help end my internal strife. It was there that I would discover there were many brothers struggling with the same issue, unable to acquire the reconciliation of sexuality and theology we were desperately seeking. No rite of passage, no guidance through puberty, no class, and no affirmation was in store for any of us in that season. Life in the closet, silenced in the "don't ask, don't tell" climate, oppressed by systems, cultures, traditions, and customs; like a blade of grass alive beneath the slab of pavement, slowly making its way through the tiny crack in weather-worn cement as it stretches toward the sun. All our lives, thus far restrained from being true to our own selves and to God.

Dealing with the world, community, or family view is one thing, but the same mentality was anchored in the Black Church, for the church comprises the makeup of the community. Being taught that God is truth, that He will love you unconditionally, and that they that worship Him must worship Him in Spirit and in truth, while at the same time being indoctrinated to believe that one is an abomination to God, can cause spiritual trauma. "Don't ask, don't tell" was also the silent mantra in the Black Church as same-gender-loving people, along with heterosexual women, remained the lesser vessels and enslaved by doctrine. Almost every reformation had someone as a member from the same-gender-loving community, more than likely silent or silenced by the culture. When one is unable to walk in truth, their worship is unable to reach its maximum potential in Christ and as a person.

Still in the midst of my struggle, in September 1986 I married a wonderful woman. Life was moving along with fervor, zest, and grace. We were both members of the military and avid blood givers. Every month as the American Red Cross mobile unit arrived, we were right there with our arms out to give. The added incentive was the day off the battalion offered for donating blood. Approximately two weeks later, while I was home from work for lunch, I answered a knock at the door. It was the mailman delivering a certified letter addressed to me from the American Red Cross. The letter stated that during screening, my blood had tested positive for the HIV antibody. Immediately life changed as I knew it.

I made my way to my commander's office and she took me to the infirmary. The diagnosis given to me by the physician was, "You have approximately six months to live, and if you survive six months, you will be bedridden the remaining days." That was it. No prescriptions. AZT was still being tested. It was plain and simple: "I have nothing that I can give or do for you to make this go away."

After weeks of being mistreated by my commanding officer, I packed my bags and drove to Walter Reed Army Medical Center. I found the Infectious Disease Clinic and requested to speak to a specialist, who placed me in protective custody for the safety of my health. I was really relieved, until I realized where I was being housed. In 1987, it had become the AIDS ward and was at its maximum capacity, housing people living with HIV/AIDS.

This was one of the most frightening and challenging times of my life. I witnessed mothers and fathers deny their children a simple hello by phone or visit, knowing these were their last days. I participated in reaching out to relatives for many, but fear and the effects of HIV/AIDS stigma kept them away. Instead, a number of us were forced to hear last words. There were even parents that were faith leaders who would not respond, would not come and visit their children. I was witness to parents arriving at the hospital to find out what was going on with their loved one, only to leave and never return. People were literally abandoning their loved ones like unwanted trash. I had never seen anything like it in my life. What kind of evil was this that would make a mother deny her own child? With all the houses of worship on every corner in Washington, DC, with all the members of the Black Church on the ward carrying a death sentence and the word had gone out. So, where were the visits from the family of faith, the representatives of God? No one came.

After months of being angry with the church and even God, after months of waiting for the church to show up, one day when I was alone in the chapel praying the Lord reminded me, "Why are you looking for the church?" he asked. "Are you not the Church, as Believer, my representative?" he continued. "Look no further!" This is the day that my ministry (gift) began to make room for me and meet a need for the Lord. I vowed to God that if I survived I would submit to His will and be a part of making a difference within this HIV/AIDS epidemic, from the pit of hell.

Where Is the Love?

HIV/AIDS profoundly challenged the Black Church's love ethic. Many houses of worship closed their doors to long-standing members and their families because of an HIV/AIDS diagnosis. After death came to the family member, funeral services and burial rights often were denied.

As fear fueled the spread of HIV, the death rate from AIDS complications also increased. One factor that exacerbated the mortality rate was the abandonment of those with HIV by family, friends, community, and even their house of worship. As soon as word of an HIV/AIDS diagnosis spread, oftentimes a person's entire support system might disappear, leaving them hopeless.

Some African American religious leaders have taken it upon themselves to "grade" sin and determine God's forgiveness. Their actions have stoked the silence on HIV in African American communities. Fear of rejection, shame, and denial also fueled divisions. For example, "recreational" drug users temporarily lulled by self-delusion distinguished themselves from drug abusers. Having an extramarital affair or multiple sex partners seemed to be "accepted"; and in some instances, it was considered a badge of honor for young men. HIV began to force some people to examine their own and their partners' past and present sexual behavior. The fact that even one unprotected sexual encounter could place a person at risk made many people uncomfortable.

Still wrestling with historically rooted issues related to discrimination, some African Americans are reluctant to acknowledge yet another issue that threatens our social "acceptability." HIV pointed the world's attention toward an aspect of life that had become twisted and negated, which at the same time was a fundamental part of African American ancestry and culture, for same-gender-loving people have always been a part of our community and houses of worship. The theology, doctrine, and tenets of the faith found themselves, in many cases, worthless when it came to practicing or living out agape. It would take losing millions of people and generations of families before truth revealed that many realized their faith was misplaced; they had fallen into worshiping and trusting their religion instead of their Lord. It's the Spirit of the Lord that brings forth life. Yet there comes a time when truth, received, will overcome the lie.

Civilian Life

After being released from Walter Reed Army Medical Center, readjusting to civilian life as a black same-gender-loving HIV-positive man would not be easy, but I had God to lean and count on, as I had every intention of upholding my vow. Unbeknownst to me, six months had long gone. Neither death nor sickness had come. It was now time to see what the end would bring for me outside of this hospital, for my faith was not strong enough at the time to believe the end was not near. I lived daily watching the demise of many as they succumbed to the very same virus that I carried within me, and I was not fully walking by faith at the time. My sight truly was impacting my walk. Yet God's grace sustained and encouraged me in spite of my doubts and fears.

I had some real decisions to make. Who would I trust to tell? Where would I live? I didn't fear rejection from my family. I just didn't want my family to witness my demise to AIDS as I had witnessed others' over the past nine months. I left Walter Reed Army Medical Center and reentered the civilian world. Life was not a skip down the Yellow Brick Road, but God's divine will and plan unfolded as I journeyed.

It took me five years to tell my mother, who was more upset about me not telling her than she was about my diagnosis. She became my number-one support system. A month later I told my next to oldest sister. She joined my support team. It took another four months before I informed my other two sisters. They all believed that my dad was not ready to hear this at the time.

In August 1995, during my family reunion's day of worship at Mount Zion Baptist Missionary Baptist Church in Laurens, South Carolina, with a packed house, the Lord sanctioned me to give my testimony. It was toward the end of service. I made my way to the front and informed my pastor that I had something that I needed to say, and I was given the microphone. As I begin to speak, preparing to make the biggest public announcement of my life, one that would probably cost me relationships and status, I found courage in the vow I gave the Lord. As the words fell from my lips, ". . . I was diagnosed with HIV," an uncomfortable quiet filled the sanctuary. I immediately moved the conversation to the fact that the diagnosis came over 10 years ago and that I praise God for his miraculous sustaining and healing power!

My testimony brought forth a praise and others began to tell other testimonies they had held in secret: a cousin with cancer and a sister in the church with leukemia. We never know what others are dealing with or going through. After the benediction, my oldest sister approached me with tears in her eyes. "How could you make that public announcement before you told your father?" she asked. "Now go to him," she said. My dad was standing over by a tree in the shade looking off into the distance. I walked over and inquired, "Are you okay, Dad?" "Are you okay?" he responded. "I am," I said. "Then let's go home," he replied.

There wasn't a great deal that changed with my presence and participation at and in church, except the growing passion and yearning from within as to what God wanted from my submission to truth. I begin to reach out to other pastors to talk about HIV/AIDS in the community, requesting their support; but doors were not open to me. HIV/AIDS was not a topic open for discussion in this season of life and ministry.

Reformations of Faith

The American Red Cross was one of the first HIV/AIDS educators in Black communities and quickly applied three lessons learned that were crucial to HIV/AIDS awareness, education, and prevention: the makeup of the messenger is crucial; the Black Church is the main entryway; and cultural competency spawns trust and renders honor.

It was in 2000, after having been one of the first African Americans in Upstate South Carolina to be certified by the American Red Cross to facilitate HIV/AIDS education for African Americans in the Black communities, that a scholarship opportunity came for me to attend the Balm in Gilead's Black Church conference on AIDS at the Kellogg Center of historical Tuskegee Institute. It was here that Spirit affirmed me, renewed my faith, endowed my purpose, and sent me forth as a warrior of God's love at a time when hate in the world, focused on the unknown and untruths surrounding HIV/AIDS, spawned a level of fear and hate the world had not witnessed since the days of Jim Crow. It was the ignorance, fear, and hate that exacerbated the deaths. (More about the Balm in Gilead later.)

Bishop Carl Bean, of Los Angeles, California, recalls a season early in his ministry where the primary assignment of the day was assisting people with AIDS to die with dignity. His ministry to the dying and some of their families brought comfort and healing to very desolate impoverished places. These strongholds of homophobia, transphobia, and hate had in some cases crippled the power to speak for one's own survival, and in other instances rendered people powerless to help their neighbor. Bishop Bean's ministry brought healing as it serviced the dying and their families with respect and love, while also confronting their vilification.

For a number of people—specifically gay, lesbian, bisexual, and transgender people—traditional theology no longer brought an appeal of a God who draws with loving kindness. Various groups of people living on the margins of society and life could not connect to mainstream faith for various reasons, but mostly because only a God of condemnation and wrath was found at the doors of most houses of worship. And during this particular season in the history of AIDS, if ever there was a time the presence of a forgiving, loving, healing God was needed, it was then. AIDS was killing people, specifically Black people, at a phenomenal rate. The death toll was exacerbated by stigma that created barriers to accessing care and challenged privacy issues. Some Black community members found courage to move beyond the boundaries of traditional theology, and thus emerged reformations of faith.

In 1982, giving the Black Church another extended arm of faith, Bishop Bean founded the Unity Fellowship Movement, a ministry for openly gay, lesbian, and bisexual African Americans. Though rejected from inclusion in the inner courts of the mainstream Black Church, Unity Fellowship Movement's call within the community to an oppressed, ostracized, and hopeless people was like that of John the Baptist's cry in the wilderness, "Repent and be ye baptized," and they came from far and wide. Unity Fellowship Movement's message was, "God is love and love is for everyone!" This message was heralded to the masses, and the rejected, ostracized, and disenfranchised came, thus receiving the love of a merciful God. Hence, faith brought new life to many.

This new movement affirmed the diversity of sexuality in community, validating the worth of the outcast by society. In particular, individuals rejected by their houses of worship now had the opportunity to experience God without external biases and hindrances. Individuals who came to the Unity Fellowship Movement learned to forgive the vilification, to heal, to love themselves, and to walk anew in faith. For many it was a life-or-death struggle to let go of the indoctrinated self-hate propagated by the belief systems that exist in many houses of worship.

As AIDS continued to lame and kill Black people, compassion touched the hearts of those made aware of Ryan White's life and death. Unfortunately, this story went virtually unnoticed in Black communities, as people felt that they had nothing in common with a young Caucasian hemophiliac. Hemophilia is not common among African Americans, and to this day many Black people do not know who Ryan White is. His death further endorsed the view that HIV/AIDS was something that affected persons other than African Americans. While this detachment was taking place, many African Americans continued to engage in risky behaviors, with increasing numbers of persons becoming HIV infected. Overcome by shame, families ostracized family members who contracted HIV. The sick were left in shelters, hospitals, and nursing homes or restricted to rooms at home. Even upon the family member's demise, fear and shame prevented families from revealing the true cause of death.

Many ministers refused to conduct funeral services for persons who had died from, or were suspected of having died from, an AIDS-related illness. More than anything else, the rejection of these family members sent a clear message: "If you become infected, you will live and die an outcast." Not even in death could one hope for salvation. The doors of the church were closed. Repentance and compassion were reserved for those sinners who found grace in the culture or standard set by the house of worship, not by their God.

Mobilization

As AIDS wiped out a generation of Black men, predominately gay and bisexual men, organizations such as Gay Men of African Descent, People of Color in Crisis, and Griot Circle, to name a few, were founded in New York City (the epicenter of the epidemic) to target Black gay men, whose infection rates were alarmingly high (as is the case today), to reduce the spread of HIV and to empower an oppressed and disenfranchised group of people.

The National Black Leadership Commission on AIDS, a policy-driven nonprofit organization working to change legislation to fight AIDS in Black communities, was founded in 1987. In 1990, the Balm in Gilead was founded, with a national mission to educate Black churches on HIV/AIDS. The Balm in Gilead's mobilization of churches and training of faith leaders opened venues for dialog within the faith community, which was crucial to the Black Church engaging in the fight against AIDS. Black churches slowly but surely began to move into a more depthful sphere of knowledge that spawned greater engagement with HIV/AIDS education and prevention. As the Balm in Gilead's national program raised awareness in the faith community, thousands of Black churches across the world developed HIV/AIDS ministries, included HIV/AIDS in their health ministry, and/or took some advocacy action.

Education was and is so needed. Without our knowledge, people living with HIV/AIDS were and are the fight's most valuable asset in combatting stigma and opening hearts to hear and receive the powerful message of prevention, along with supporting the care for people living with HIV/AIDS. I didn't know where this journey of faith was taking me. I just knew that I wanting to live and God's grace had granted my prayers. I made a vow, and I can't take it back.

A Calling

I had followed the lead of the Lord, which guided my footsteps. I told my pastor that I had been called to the ministry by God, and I graduated from the seminary, volunteering at the only long-term care facility in South Carolina for people living with HIV/AIDS. During my senior year as a student, I was required to have 400 hours of preaching and teaching in a local assembly. That was not doable at the church God had now moved me to, Evangelical House of God in Taylors, South Carolina. There were 13 ministers, not counting myself. There was no space for that kind of time. It was here that God poured out his healing love upon me, the place where the prophetic word of God endowed me and raised me up. It was in this sacred place that Bishop James Dawkins, led by the Lord, licensed me to preach the gospel of Jesus Christ. In his obedience he paid a major price, as he was ridiculed among his peers and confronted by his own. Yet, he knew in his spirit what God wanted. The Lord used this great man of God to give me beauty for ashes as I was resurrected from the dead in the Black Church, after having come to him as I was—broken and in need of another dimension of God. He provided me God's unconditional love, looking beyond any fault and meeting me at my point of need.

The pastor of Tabernacle Baptist Church offered me the opportunity to come assist him in starting his HIV/AIDS ministry and complete the 400 hours I needed to graduate. All was going well. The people seemed to really love me. There was even a good reception after he allowed me to share my testimony. As usual, things were not as they seemed. I later discovered the petition started by a deacon, stating that my HIV status defiled the pulpit. It requested that I not be dismissed, only not allowed to sit in the pulpit. This situation was resolved by me humbling myself, pleading with the pastor not to contest, and doing what I had been sent there to do. I understood that my presence was all the education some people needed, in terms of where they were, concerning HIV/AIDS education, prevention, care, and ministry.

Engagement

A number of cutting-edge Black churches began to engage the plight of AIDS in Black communities much earlier than most realize and have continued to do consistently phenomenal work with their constituents and the broader community to prevent the spread of HIV and end AIDS. Many have been featured and honored by the Balm in Gilead, the National Black Leadership Commission on AIDS, departments of health, and/or other entities for their efforts. Some churches have been working tirelessly in their communities and will never be known to the masses. But if truth be known, collectively the Black Church has always lagged behind in outpouring love, extending grace, and applying mercy when engaging HIV/AIDS. Yet, God always has a remnant working on his behalf.

But when one comprehends the cultural and historical factors involved, the fear that accompanies ignorance, the unknowns about HIV/AIDS, the way and the time the Black community was informed and the actions taken by authorities to assist, the reluctance and lack of engagement on the part of the Black community and the Black Church is to some degree understandable. Consider that global mobility was considered the principle facilitator of HIV. Other theories regarding the spread of HIV pointed to the use of unsterilized needles or biological warfare. Regardless of the theoretical route, they all led to Africa. Whether intentional or not, the manner in which these theories were expressed seemed to further vilify dark-skinned people of African descent, whose image was already distorted among many. Further, close to this time frame there was an acknowledgement of the atrocity of the Tuskegee syphilis experiment. African Americans were distrustful, at best, of any government initiative that attributed the origin of HIV to them. Circumstances like these increased Blacks' nonparticipation in reaction to health guidance offered by the government.

Ultimately, we see the Lord raising up a remnant of workers through various nonprofit entities to aid in assisting the Black Church to become more aware of and educated about HIV. Many Black churches began forming their own nonprofit entities and providing services for HIV/AIDS. Today, we have faith-based initiatives in which involvement of religious leaders and organizations in HIV/AIDS prevention have a major impact.

Gratitude

At the same time, I must say that I am grateful for love. Love is the only thing that overcomes ALL things. Thank God my family, being active members of the Black Church, were able to maintain their love ethic afforded through their faith. They loved and cared for me beyond their fears, doubts, and religious upbringing. They allowed God to be God, for it's the Spirit of God that will lead us into all truths about life, love, and sexuality. Without my family, including my church family, I honestly don't know if I would be here, particularly when I began antiretrovirals in 1995. The initial side effects were horrible. There were days that I just didn't want to go through with it. It was my mother saying, "You want me to come in there and make you take that medicine?" that encouraged my heart. It was my sister crying, sleeping, and praying at the foot of my bed those initial two weeks of starting medication that gave me the support I needed to get through to the other side. It was the Black Church in my life, on my journey, that made sure there was a place at the table for me. Thus, the work through my ministry of the Black Church continues. Until we are all free, no one is free.

No One Is Coming to Save Us

While more African Americans were facing the grim reality of HIV infection in their community and beginning to educate themselves about the disease, more needed to be done to raise awareness and change behaviors. The effectiveness of HIV prevention education has been demonstrated in numerous communities, populations, and countries. HIV/AIDS prevention works. But it was necessary that Black churches engage the process to change future outcomes for Black people. Local community residents would need to take the lead and not depend on state or federal governments to sanction their efforts to establish prevention education. The saying remains true: "No one is coming to save us [Black people]. We must save ourselves."

To raise awareness, concerned individuals began advertising campaigns, held conferences, and started nationwide initiatives. Billboards depicting African American couples stressed the need for safer sex practices, much to the dismay of some church leaders who petitioned to have them removed. These billboards did not emphasize values that the Black Church community wished to promote—such as abstinence and fidelity—and were viewed as encouraging promiscuity. The advertising campaigns sought to communicate with people where they were, rather than where religious leaders felt they should be.

Even in the face of increasing numbers of congregants becoming infected and affected, even with the phenomenal work the Balm in Gilead was doing, African American communities of faith, generally speaking, persisted in their refusal to collectively acknowledge the severity of HIV infection nationwide. It seemed easier to condemn than to acknowledge the limitations of their compassion. It was almost as if the Black Church was willing to let an entire group of people suffer and die without providing them with any of the support made available to the homeless, the poor, and the otherwise infirm. Many believe that it was this denial that was responsible for increasing the spread of the disease. They felt that had HIV been addressed from the outset, it would not have reached epidemic proportions within this sector of society.

The NAACP, the US Surgeon General, the Centers for Disease Control, the Reverend Jesse Jackson, and Kweisi Mfume, along with other noted African American leaders and organizations, attempted to bring the seriousness of HIV infection to the forefront in the African American community. Their efforts drew media attention, but their message was not heeded by those most affected and most at risk, African Americans. Many African Americans, despite these and many other national efforts, did not and still do not feel that HIV should concern them. Despite the declaration made by former President Clinton that HIV infection was now at epidemic proportions among African Americans, national prevention efforts were not reaching community residents where it was most needed—at the grassroots level.

Preventive education regarding HIV in these communities was not nearly as pervasive as it should have been. While some experts attempted to correlate socioeconomics and the spread of HIV among African Americans, the virus spread so rapidly that it clearly defied socioeconomic, ethnic, and religious boundaries. African Americans are not genetically predisposed to HIV; rather, it was often an issue of being uninformed and, therefore, unable to alter behavior that places individuals at risk. Preventive education, a proven vehicle to address this issue, did not reach far enough into the general population.

More Black churches were becoming involved in AIDS advocacy and education, but more needed to join the ranks of the fight. For the purpose of expository learning and a healing of a people, the Balm in Gilead hosted its Third Annual Black Church HIV/ADS Training Institute, May 22–24, 2001, at Tuskegee University to examine the impact HIV/AIDS had on Black people and the role that members of faith-based institutions must play in AIDS prevention, treatment, and care. Black clergy came from all across the country. Their presence spoke care. Their compassionate engagement revealed passionate concern. After returning from the training institute at the Kellogg Center, we were able to return to Upstate South Carolina and mobilize over 30 churches to implement and participate in ongoing HIV/AIDS education and prevention activities.

In October 2007, Bishop T. D. Jakes, CEO of the Potter's House of Dallas, Texas, joined with Reverend Dr. Calvin O. Butts III, chair of the National Black Leadership Commission on AIDS National Conclave on HIV/AIDS Policy for Black Clergy, to partner with the National Medical Association, the Congressional Black Caucus Health Brain Trust, the National Conference of Black Mayors, the National Caucus of Black State Legislators, and the New York community. The Conclave convened a public policy summit with over 150 Black leaders that included senior members of Congress and over 80 clergy representing the Black Church. The purpose of the gathering was to create a clergy-led plan of action that would address the state of emergency in the Black community regarding HIV/AIDS prevention, treatment, and care across the nation.

The two-day summit concluded with participants issuing a paper that again cited the devastating toll of the US HIV/AIDS epidemic on Black America, and they proposed several recommendations that targeted funding in an effort to form a comprehensive response that addressed the multiple challenges posed by the AIDS-driven public health crisis. All leaders in attendance were to return to their communities and districts, staying accountable to their constituents in maintaining the plan of action.

Transformation Through Faith and Education

The foundation of the faith-based approach is faith and education. Historically, faith and education have sustained African Americans through difficult periods and have figured prominently in helping to overcome challenging circumstances. Faith is the key ingredient in spiritual transformation, and education is the conduit through which people prepare for life's beckoning "opportunities."

In the struggle against HIV/AIDS, the Black Church can integrate faith and education in ways that help individuals move from information to transformation amid the trials and triumphs of life. Working independently and collaboratively, today's Black churches can use their tremendous resources to overcome the barriers of denial, complacency and ignorance, and to usher in a new day of victory over the scourge of HIV/AIDS. As we continue into the 21st century, every ministry needs to embrace HIV education, prevention, and care so that we may stop the spread of HIV and end AIDS in Black communities.

Having engaged Black churches across this country as a minister, preacher, pastor, and HIV/AIDS educator and activist, I am a living witness that prevention works. Working with Black churches throughout South Carolina during 1996 through 2002, conducting outreach and education for the American Red Cross and Project Care, I have seen HIV/AIDS education and prevention work. As a worker with National Train the Trainer for the Interdenominational Theological Center "Affirming a Future with Hope: HIV & Substance Abuse Prevention for African American Communities of Faith," working with churches nationally, I am a witness that HIV/AIDS education and prevention work. As a staff member of the Balm in Gilead working with Black churches across the nation to educate and impact the fight against HIV/AIDS, I have seen HIV/AIDS education and prevention work. Working with communities of faith nationally through the African American Capacity Building Initiative of Harm Reduction Coalition, I know HIV/AIDS prevention and education work, if you work it.

Finding My Calling in Hell
My Journey Through the Early Years of AIDS

RAYFORD KYTLE

I LIVED IN New York City from May 1975 until December 1980. I was
working full time, but what I remember most was the music, the dancing,
the drugs, and the sex. Am I ashamed that I squandered my youth? Not at
all. Having been suffocated, shrouded, and nearly buried by my upbringing,
I was gasping for air. It's a wonder I survived it.

Beginning in the eighth grade in Richmond, Virginia, in 1958, homophobia was psychologically and emotionally drummed into me. As I began to
realize I was attracted to other boys, there were no social structures to
help me meet others like me and slowly develop mutual affection and respect. Assumed to be heterosexual, I was introduced to girls through
family, friends, church socials, school dances, and parties. I dated lots of
beautiful, smart, and funny girls. Many of them are still close friends. First
date, first kiss, falling in love for the first time—I knew from movies what
they were supposed to be like. I tried to act them out. What I didn't know,
however, what my classmates talked about all the time, was what it felt like
to experience those events under the influence of raging hormones. Girls
thought I was so "nice," such a gentleman, so different from the other boys
who pawed at them, trying to hide or showing off their erections. It was easy
to be a gentleman because my hormones were gay and I was spending all the
psychic energy I could muster to extinguish them.

Prayer and a series of therapists helped me to bury the internal gyroscope
of my feelings for 14 years. I started seeing a psychiatrist the summer before
my senior year in high school. I had read that "homosexual tendencies"
could be "cured" if the patient really wanted to be. He said I was just going
through a phase.

The Civil Rights and anti–Vietnam War movements shattered my respect for societal homophobia. The people who blew up Sunday schools in Alabama and napalmed children in Vietnam were the same people who condemned homosexuality.

While visiting a close friend from college, who was in medical school at the University of Virginia, I found out that he was gay. He and his friends showed me that gay people could be successful, respected, contributing members of society. When I returned to William and Mary, where I was getting a master's degree in sociology, I bought some marijuana for the first time. Stoned, alone in my apartment, I allowed my fantasies to float over the walls I had built to contain them. I allowed myself to see and accept that I was gay and that there was no reason to be ashamed about it. That night I was able to find myself and begin to trust my feelings and let them guide me. I felt like my life was beginning.

I wanted to get away from the people, the culture, and the stereotypes that had beaten me down. I still carried wounds from high school: feeling left out and despised, an emasculated wimp. Once I'd accepted and respected myself, I wanted to stand up tall in the sunlight, hold my head high, and look people in the eye—as wholesome as baseball and apple pie. I no longer had anything to hide. I wanted to be what I thought of as masculine: brave, rugged, and straightforward. I wanted to face life with all my resources, including my sexuality. I wanted men to endorse me as fully human, acceptable, and attractive—finally, to be one of the guys.

Once I escaped the gauntlet of homophobia, my sexuality overflowed like lava. Sex wasn't just physical pleasure, even when accompanied by affection. It was also political, healing, and cathartic: a thrilling sensation of rebellion, winning, and freedom. It was a kick in the groin to all those who had told me I was sick and evil because of who I loved.

One weekend in Manhattan convinced me that was where I needed to be. I moved there in summer 1975, when gay people were building skyscrapers of liberation.

I was torn between the desire to help establish a new social order—peace and justice for everyone, including gay people—on the one hand and the desire to explore my sexuality and celebrate my rebirth on the other. The trick was to find a balance.

What remained of my Presbyterian upbringing was a sense that everyone has a "calling," a way to use all their talents and resources to help make the world a better place. I had been trying to obliterate my deepest feelings for so long, I had no idea what my "calling" might be. Once I'd moved to Manhattan, I couldn't imagine leaving, even though the job market was ferociously competitive. Instead of rationally navigating a career that would challenge me and develop all my resources, I took the first job I could find that seemed to be focused on doing good.

I worked as a claims representative for Social Security Supplemental Security Income (SSI) benefits in Harlem. SSI provides minimal income and Medicaid to elderly, blind, and disabled people whose work history doesn't qualify them for a regular Social Security (SSA) benefit above the poverty line. Although SSI clients were frequently mentally ill, we received no special training in how to elicit information from them. I felt like I worked in the tortured world of the wretched of the earth. Being kind to the clients was just good enough to justify my getting stoned and escaping into the gay party circuit and the cultural feast of the city nearly every waking hour away from work.

In winter 1976, I started seeing George, the business manager for a small gay travel and catering company. George took me behind the velvet rope of New York's Dionysian gay life. He took me to Flamingo, the premier private gay disco, where we danced on Saturday nights; to the Everard baths where the hottest guys went; to the 23rd Street YMCA, where we worked out, socialized and cruised the sauna; and to fabulous parties. From the end of March until mid-September, we spent weekends on "The Island"—The Pines, an idyllic gay resort community on Fire Island for the rich, the successful, the brilliant, and the beautiful.

In summer 1978, I read *Dancer from the Dance* by Andrew Holleran and *Faggots* by Larry Kramer. Both books conveyed disenchantment with the life I was living, expressing a yearning to heal the rift between ephemeral eroticism and faithful friendship. Both called for gay people to use our new freedom to do something more than create pleasure palaces in our ghettos. Both deserve credit for being written before AIDS showed that their messages were a matter of life and death. Those books helped me to see that I was neglecting a big part of who I was and who I wanted to become. I hadn't found the right balance between working to make things better and seeking pleasure.

I told a friend that I didn't feel good about my life. He sent me to a great lesbian therapist, Gloria Donadello, who said I needed to *do* something that would make me feel better about myself. She told me about SAGE, an organization just forming to provide social services to gay and lesbian elders. I attended organizational meetings, cowrote their first procedures manual, and served on their first board of directors. After a year or so, however, I felt it was taking too much of my free time. I felt pulled back into the circuit of sex, drugs, and disco. Many years later, I realized that I was addicted. Sex became a panacea—an escape, both from the cutthroat competition for power and money all around me, as well as from the work required to make the world a better place. I didn't want to fight back or compete that way, any more than I had wanted to play football in the eighth grade. I thought fierce competition diminished the possibly of male intimacy that I craved. My self-esteem, which had soared when I started my life as a gay man, was eroding.

Internalized homophobia has more layers than pastry dough, and it takes a lifetime to overcome, if ever. When I felt guilty, worthless, and overwhelmed, I just got stoned and grabbed a taxi to the baths, where, for a time, I could feel artificially happy. At the baths, I didn't have to introduce myself, establish my socioeconomic status, or unload any baggage. At the baths, it just took a moment to lock eyes; the chemistry was either there or it wasn't. At the baths, I could feel like a million bucks. Sexual power, however, was the only currency that made me feel flush.

George moved to San Francisco and I met Jon at Flamingo in March 1979. Jon was a professional fundraiser whose disposable income was nearly twice the amount of mine. We split most costs between us, but Jon paid for our shares at The Pines.

As we were packing up to leave The Island, in September 1979, Jon told me that he hadn't felt quite right for about a year. By then I was in love with him and I didn't get angry with him for not telling me sooner. He suggested we both get tested for mononucleosis. I began a series of tests that ended a year later at Sloan-Kettering. The diagnosis was that I had an unidentifiable low-grade virus. During that year, as my doctor advised, I had slowed down my extramural sexual activity and stayed away from the baths. In the end, however, all the doctors I saw told me to just live my life as I had been doing before all the tests.

When he got a great job offer in Washington, DC, Jon wanted me to come with him, and after five years in New York City, I was ready to leave. I was able to transfer to a Social Security office in a tony neighborhood just a few minutes' walk from where we were living. The applicants' lives, however, were the same as in New York.

When the first article about a new gay disease appeared in the *New York Times* in June 1981, I telephoned my hematologist at Sloan-Kettering. He said, "Don't worry, we checked for that."

Living in Washington, Jon and I didn't notice people disappearing the way we would have if we'd still been living in New York. But every time we visited New York, we would run into friends who'd started having symptoms of the new virus. When someone we'd known on The Island became sick, disfigured, or terminal, they stopped coming out on weekends and it was possible—assuming they weren't close friends—to pretend that nothing had changed. A stigma became attached to the "gay virus," even among gay people.

Jon and I took the HIV test the first chance we got, at the National Institutes of Health, in June 1984. That September, after a frenzied summer, our tests came back positive. It was no surprise. Jon and I agreed that if one of us got sick, the other would take care of him.

When we found out we were both HIV positive, we agreed to follow the CDC's guidelines and reduced the number of people we were sleeping with, stopped going to the baths, and always used condoms. I decided that sexual intimacy was more important than specific sexual acts.

A few months after our pledge, when Jon emptied his pockets, I noticed a matchbook from a bath house in Los Angeles. When I confronted him, Jon said, "I'm going out with my boots on."

By 1985 Jon and I had been together for six years. One gorgeous Saturday at The Pines, Jon said he felt like he had the flu and that he needed to go home. His fever spiked and I took him to the emergency room at George Washington University Hospital, where he was diagnosed with *Pneumocystis* pneumonia. "It's a death sentence, isn't it?" he asked. It was. There were drugs that could treat the symptomatic diseases associated with it, but there was nothing to treat the underlying virus destroying his immune system.

Jon was ashamed that he had AIDS, and he didn't even want any of our friends to know he was sick. His good looks disappeared as he got hollowed out, thin, and frail. As he got sicker and bedridden, taking care of him became a full-time job. We couldn't afford qualified people to stay with him 24–7. One day I dropped him trying to clean him up, and I just gave up. I called 911. He was furious that I was sending him back to the hospital. He had every reason to hate it. Every time he went, they put what amounted to a skull and crossbones on his door and treated him like a leper. His doctor didn't respect our relationship.

Eventually, however, when I came to see him, he told me that he realized that I was trying to take care of him the best I could. He said that he had dreamed he was in a prison yard and he looked up and saw me sailing over the wall in a hot air balloon, throwing him a rope. He said he hadn't really loved me before, but he loved me now. Those words were bittersweet, coming so late; but still, they were a magnificent gift. I try to remember them when I feel guilty that I didn't do a better job of caring for him.

Jon developed dementia in the hospital and began having delusions. He was starting to lose his sight and hearing. He became so sensitive to touch that when I tried to hold his hand he recoiled. I had promised him that I would make sure he was not in pain. I lost confidence in his doctor and the hospital.

I'd heard wonderful things about the Washington Home and Hospice. I called and made an appointment and met with two hospice nurses and a physician who was an expert in pain management. They accepted Jon into the hospice that afternoon and he died that night.

I had a gathering at our apartment in memory of Jon. All our friends asked me why I hadn't been in touch with them. I just told them that was the way Jon wanted it. I went to New York and had a small gathering at a friend's apartment. The next day, he drove me to Sayville, the idyllic little town on Long Island where Jon was born and grew up, and where we caught the ferry to The Pines. I put some rose petals in the water, along with his ashes, so that they would float toward the place where he'd been the happiest.

So many people had to tell their parents not only were they gay but they had AIDS—sometimes being condemned and abandoned by them. I was very lucky. Dad would send Jon a bottle of Old Spice at Christmas, but he had never acknowledged we were anything more than friends. Then, over the Thanksgiving holiday in 1985, Dad and I went for a walk. He suddenly said, "Son, so Jon is sick?" I said, "Yeah, Dad, he is. In fact, he's going to die," and I just broke down. Dad said, "Oh son, I'm so sorry. I remember what it felt like when your mother died." Dad and I never felt loved by anyone more than her. From that moment until he died, 15 years later, we became as close as we had been when I was four and we would dress up for the YMCA's Indian Guides as Big and Little Chief Red Feather.

After Jon died, I began to focus on how many of our friends were sick and dying. Sometimes I would try to contact old friends I hadn't been in touch with for a while, and I'd find out they had died and no one had let me know. In summer 1978, George and I had been in a small house on the ocean at The Pines. There were eight of us. All died of AIDS except me.

My T-cell count remained above 500, which was considered relatively healthy, and my doctor didn't put me on AZT right away. I read everything I could find about AIDS and experimental anti-HIV drug trials. I signed up for the trials as fast as I could.

Later, in 1992, just as my T-cell count dipped below 200, classifying me as having "full blown" AIDS, a nutritionist I'd been seeing, Lark Lands, told me about interleukin-2, which elevated the immune system and was in clinical trials at NIH. I volunteered but was told I'd have to have my gall bladder removed. I did but then was randomized into the control group. I would have to wait six months to get the drug. Lark told me that Dr. Frank Bruni, in private practice, was always on the cutting edge of AIDS treatments, and he was providing the drug to his patients. I had to pay for it and it was expensive, but his office said they would try to get Blue Cross to pay for it and I didn't have to pay anything until they worked things out with Blue Cross. Eventually, I ended up owing Blue Cross a lot of money. I had to file for bankruptcy, but the treatment had kept me healthy until the life-saving cocktail of highly active anti-retroviral treatments (HAART) became available in 1996.

I began speaking publicly about my experience with HIV after Jon died. I signed up with the Speakers Bureau for the National Association of People with AIDS. The first time I spoke was to the staff at George Washington (GW) Hospital. Someone in the audience asked me why I'd stayed with Jon, considering how he had treated me. The question just threw me. I wondered if a spouse would have been asked that question.

AIDS patients began to apply for benefits at my Social Security office about the time that Jon got sick, in June 1985. Nearly all of them were gay men. AIDS stigma and the fear of contagion were rampant, along with homophobia. Pat Robertson and Jesse Helms were quoted in the press saying that God's wrath was descending on perverts who deserved what they got. Eddie Murphy made jokes about AIDS patients on his HBO special. President Reagan didn't even utter the word "AIDS" until September 1985, by which time nearly 23,000 Americans, mostly gay Americans, had been diagnosed with AIDS and well over 12,000 had died from it. My brother didn't want me to touch his children. I couldn't really blame him; back then no one knew exactly how the virus could be transmitted.

At work, I overheard other claims representatives' interactions with AIDS patients, who were usually exhausted from the trip to the office and the long wait in the reception area that was typically filled with homeless, mentally ill people. The stench was sometimes unbearable. Claimants often had colds or flu that were easily transmitted to people with no immune systems. The AIDS patients were emaciated, disfigured, and bitter. I could see and hear that some of the other claims representatives cut them no slack. If AIDS patients were rude to them, the claims representatives gave it right back.

I felt burned out after 10 years of trying to quickly force miserable, chaotic lives into boxes on government forms, helping people whose lives seemed so disconnected from mine. Many of them resented me, understandably, and I don't recall anyone ever expressing appreciation for what I was doing.

Then suddenly there were people like me across my desk, and they were dying from an illness I had. I could imagine the additional ordeals and indignities they were facing—possibly abandoned by their lovers and families, unable to work, worrying about food and rent money, frequently having to deal with bureaucrats who had little sympathy for them, if not contempt. Being able to help people I understood and related to, people who could so easily be my friends, or be me, lifted my spirits instead of depressing me.

In 1986, I volunteered to take both SSI and SSA disability applications from all AIDS applicants in my office (many of the AIDS applicants had sufficient work history to qualify for some regular Social Security disability benefits). Other Social Security offices were happy to send AIDS cases somewhere else, so I began to handle all the SSI/SSA AIDS applications for the Metro Washington, DC area, including the Virginia and Maryland suburbs.

I began to work over the phone with the Washington, DC, Disability Determinations Service (DDS) and learned exactly what documentation was needed to approve an AIDS application. Proof of having any one of a number of opportunistic infections qualified a person for "presumptive" disability, meaning immediate payment and Medicaid.

Whitman Walker Clinic, the gay men's clinic that had been so helpful to me during Jon's illness, asked me if there was some way that I could help them with their large caseload of people with AIDS. I began training volunteers to complete all the paperwork for an application prior to coming into the office, including documentation of the earliest onset of their qualifying illnesses, which could cover SSA's five-month waiting period and get immediate payment. Sometimes this entitled them to substantial back payments of their SSA disability benefits. Eventually, I was able to get the DDS to cooperate with SSI/SSA so that claims could be approved the same day we received the application, enabling dying AIDS patients to get out of the hospital to come home to die.

I don't remember ever feeling any gratitude from applicants with other disabilities, and I never expected to. I knew I hadn't done much to alleviate their misery. But it was very different with AIDS applicants. I remember a distinguished Army general I interviewed for SSI for his gay son, who had progressive multifocal leukoencephalopathy, one of the cruelest of the AIDS-related opportunistic infections. I could see how hard it was for him to talk about his son, who had made jewelry for a living and never paid Social Security. I imagined what a difficult relationship they must have had. He later wrote a letter to the office manager commending me for the way I had treated him and the efficiency of my work.

One day a woman came in to apply for her son who had AIDS. As she described him I realized he was someone I knew from the New York circuit.

I told his mother and she was so relieved to have found a bureaucrat who knew firsthand what she and her son were going through. She invited me over to her apartment to see her son, and after he died she and I remained friends until her death, 10 years later.

I realized that in the midst of all the suffering and dying brought on by AIDS, I had found my calling. My early weak attempt to do good had prepared me to use the skills I'd learned—along with my heart and soul—to make what seemed to be a significant contribution to the nightmarish battle going on all around me. My job gave me a sense of agency during a time when there was so little anyone could do to help. I felt my work life integrate with my personal life. Every day I came home knowing I had done something to help someone I could relate to, someone like me. I wasn't helping many people with AIDS who were different from me—the women and babies in Africa, for instance, who were usually referred to as "innocent victims." I wasn't risking my job or putting my life on the line, fighting for lifesaving meds, like activists I knew in New York. I was only comforting the dying—and being paid for it, with top-notch health insurance and a pension. Still, it felt good to know that I was doing it well.

I became known and respected by many in the DC gay community. I was interviewed and honored, and in December 1988, I was promoted to a job in the press office of the assistant secretary for health (OASH) at the Department of Health and Human Services. The assistant secretary for health was the head of the Public Health Service, which at that time comprised eight agencies, including the National Institutes of Health, the Food and Drug Administration, and the Centers for Disease Control. OASH was where federal AIDS policy was made. I felt I was moving closer to the power to really make a difference.

Reading now about those early years of AIDS, I think I am on maybe the B-list of those who helped to ease the pain it caused and worked to end it, at least in Washington, DC. But I've been fortunate in many ways, chief among them to have worked among and for people who supported me as a gay man with AIDS. I've also had the luxury of access to excellent health insurance; to Doug Ward and other top-tier doctors and research teams, many of whom are gay and all of whom are empathetic; and of great gay therapists—one in particular, Gary Raymond. He has helped me to understand that each of us travels their own path, through the thicket of their unique experiences with their unique genes and resources.

We are told in America that there are only winners and losers, first prize or nothing to write home about. Perhaps it serves a purpose to make people try their hardest. But it can be intimidating, too, so that some people give up trying. Most people, however, like me, are somewhere in the middle and will be forgotten except by those who love them. Even so, small contributions matter; intention matters. Each of us does what we can, putting our best selves and our best efforts out there, sharing what love and compassion we can muster, hoping that it will create ripples that go from one person to the next forever. I try to tell myself that's okay, and most of the time it is.

What Did You Learn, Dorothy?

ROBERT LOVE

M Y NAME IS ROBERT LOVE. I moved to San Francisco in 1970, three months after I turned 18, to live with someone with whom I was having a long-distance relationship. We were together for a few years while I was going to school. I was employed as a nurseryman in the East Bay and commuted to work with a good friend of mine who lived in The City and also worked at the nursery. One of my favorite memories of my friend is that he would, on a weekly basis, sidle up to me mid-day at the nursery and whisper, "I think I need a beauty treatment. Let's go to Elizabeth Arden's tonight." Elizabeth Arden was his code name for his favorite bathhouse.

In the mid-1970s, in the newly established gay neighborhood in San Francisco, the Castro, there was a local watering hole called the Corner Grocery Bar that was known for playing opera on the jukebox and having live recitals on weekends. Since opera was (and still is) my passion, I would go to the bar two or three times a week to listen to and discuss opera. I became good friends with all the bartenders and we would meet every Monday morning, along with three other friends, at the Café Flor in the Castro. There were seven of us in our group. Three of my buddies were from the bar and the other three were hairdressers. We all had Mondays off and would meet at the Café Flor and play dominoes. We were a tight group of twenty-somethings and, I admit, we were all very sexually active.

In 1976, I met and set up housekeeping with James. We were together for 13 years and were relatively monogamous during our time together.

Sometime in the 1980s, a good friend who was a veterinarian began sharing his concern about a mysterious illness affecting many of his friends. His concern grew to the point where he and other members of the community began setting up information tables at various bathhouses to warn patrons about this illness. At the same time, we began to hear in the news about this illness outside of the gay community. It was becoming a major concern among our friends. My veterinarian friend became increasingly active in efforts to reach out to the community. Sadly, he was the first of my friends who died from the disease. It was shocking for all of us to witness his deterioration and how he wasted away. This was the beginning of losing each of my friends from the Café Flor to AIDS.

Most of the guys moved north of The City to the Russian River area to get away from the plague and to take care of themselves and their partners. Over the next decade, the churches, the mortuary, and the Guerneville Cemetery became very familiar to all of us. I was a pallbearer for all six of my friends, laying them to rest in the cemetery.

A poignant note to these funerals was that at the end of each service we played the closing aria from the American opera *The Ballad of Baby Doe* by Douglas Moore. I had introduced this opera to everyone at the Corner Grocery Bar and it was a favorite among my friends. The closing lines of the opera are sung by the title character as she stands alone in the snow at the mouth of the silver mine she was told to hold onto by her late husband: "As our earthly eyes grow dim, still the old song will be sung. I will change along with him so that both are ever young, ever young." To this day, it's very difficult for me to hear that aria.

James and I became very concerned regarding this mysterious disease, not to mention being concerned about our own health. In retrospect, I imagine the combination of being monogamous, along with my own sexual preferences, kept us relatively isolated from the infection. Oral sex has always been my preference and anything more intimate was usually reserved by me for those with whom I was having a long-term relationship. However, so little was known about the disease that everyone became paranoid if they had something as simple as a cold. I recall coming down with what turned out to be the flu. I noticed that the lymph nodes on my neck were slightly swollen and by the time I was able to see my physician I was completely convinced that I was infected. My physician reassured me that the state of my lymph nodes was nothing compared to what he had seen in men who were infected with HIV and had full-blown AIDS. He did insist that I get tested for HIV and my relief from learning that I was negative was profound.

We were living in the Cow Hollow neighborhood of The City at the time. Our landlord owned a gay retreat up in the Russian River area. He eventually also became infected. At that time, researchers from the University of California Medical Center were canvassing neighborhoods where cases of

AIDS had been reported. One evening a gentleman showed up, identified himself as one of the researchers, and asked if I might be interested in participating in a study about this new, mysterious disease. I felt participating in such a study was a small way of helping to discover the cause of the disease.

This began a 10-year collaboration with UCMC in which I would go to either the hospital on Parnassus Avenue or to San Francisco General Hospital every six months to answer a plethora of questions and for them to take blood samples and give a physical exam. To this day, I have never received so much attention from doctors and researchers concerning my health. The questionnaires and interviews would take almost two hours to complete. I received quite the education from these questions about drugs and sexual practices that I had no idea ever existed.

I believe that the people leading the research were pleased to have someone in their study that was, and continued to be, HIV negative for the duration of the study. I was told that my blood was extensively researched and was always tested for any trace of HIV whenever a new sample was drawn.

Eventually, the research staff became good friends. After the AIDS study ended, I was asked to continue being a participant in a men's anal cancer study.

Going to SF General Hospital was always a sobering experience, especially as the disease spread and the AIDS ward began to have more and more patients. I think the absolute worst manifestation of the disease was the Kaposi's sarcoma lesions that would appear on the arms and hands and faces of the patients infected with HIV. It was shocking to be at the theater or at a store and glance over at someone with those hideous black spots on their face and realize how little time they had left. It felt even more shocking and tragic when you saw these lesions appear on your friends.

James and I felt we had to do something, so we both signed up as volunteers with the Shanti Project—an organization dedicated to enhancing the quality of life of persons living with life-threatening or chronic illnesses—and offered our help. James signed up as an emotional support volunteer. Given my practical nature, I signed up for practical support, which included offering to help clean the client's home, taking them shopping, doing laundry, etc.

Over the next eight years I had about a dozen different clients, all of whom I stayed with until their passing. My strongest memory is spending hour upon hour in laundromats washing sheets and bed linens because of the ever-present diarrhea these men experienced. I used to have bags and bags of quarters in my truck in order to run the machines. And one needed to be somewhat circumspect because people were so paranoid at the time about the disease and the sight of someone washing all those sheets would cause angry questioning by the other patrons at the laundromat as to why I was washing so many sheets and where they came from. I would usually lie and tell people I worked at a convalescent home and our machine was broken.

Eventually, James and I decided we should participate with Shanti in another form, so we enrolled at the National Holistic Institute, where we got our massage certificates. James specialized in shiatsu and relaxation techniques and I focused more on lymphatic massage. We would take our tables to the various clients and offer them massage.

In time, however, we both realized we were burning ourselves out and we needed to pull back from our volunteer efforts to maintain our sanity. Also, more and better treatment came along, so many of the practical support activities we had been performing were no longer needed.

Looking back, I have very strong memories of these remarkable men who died from this disease. I was always amazed how strong and accepting of their fate they were. One of my favorite clients, who loved to cook, would ask me to take him shopping in his wheelchair and he would buy the most wonderful foods and take them home and make lavish meals for his friends, regardless of the fact that he could hardly walk. I remember the day when he finally had to have an in-house caretaker. I walked into his kitchen where he had the caretaker looking through his cookbooks so that she could cook and serve a big dinner for his friends. I also marveled at his laissez-faire attitude about his fate when his weight plummeted to 100 pounds. He said, "Well, 10 more pounds and I'll be dead. Everyone knows, if you have AIDS, when you reach 90 pounds its checkout time."

There are so many sad and painful memories that still make me angry to this day. James had two clients, both very shy, quiet, and sweet young men who were reaching the end of their lives. They were completely devoted to each other and rarely went anywhere without the other. When one of the men died, his mother and sister came over from Sweden. His mother was a born-again Christian and completely intolerant of gay people. Since the house they were living in was in her son's name, she threw his partner out in the street and claimed the house and the belongings as hers. The partner went to live in a shelter and a week later took his own life by ingesting an overdose of the painkillers that were prescribed to him and his partner.

I remember the mother of one of my clients whom I would call on a weekly basis to inform her of the status of her son's health because he was very reluctant to tell her what was going on. He would tell his mom to "ask

Robert." She lived in a small, rural Georgia town. When her son eventually passed away, she asked that I come and visit her if I had a chance. She said, "Robert, you took care of my boy and now you are my boy." I did go visit her in Georgia and I will always remember her taking me aside before being introduced to her friends and family. She said, "Please don't tell anyone what my son died from. They don't understand." She passed away a few years later, but to this day I am still deeply saddened that this poor woman had no one in her life with whom she could share the facts about her son's life and death. The isolation and loneliness she experienced from her son's death were so obvious. I told her friends that her son had died from cancer.

There are so many other stories that I could share. I recall one of the more interesting conversations I had with my grandmother who passed away a few years ago at the age of 102. When the disease was at its strongest and I was losing so many friends, she had reached the age where she was losing her friends and contemporaries from old age. She was so angry about what I was going through. She said, "It's bad enough that a person has to experience losing all their friends and loved ones once in their lives. You are going to have to experience it twice. It's not fair."

I sometimes think that I have become somewhat jaded about death and disease. I admit that I can no longer feel the depth of emotion about those close to me dying as I once did 30 years ago. Perhaps this is normal. I cannot say I feel somehow blessed that I was never infected with the virus. The sense of loss and sadness I feel whenever I think of everyone that I know who died way too young certainly outweighs any feelings of luck or blessings received from not being infected.

I am now 64 years old and very happily married to a wonderful man. I only wish that he could have met all those amazing friends of mine who died from the disease.

A closing story. There are few things about AIDS that bothered me more when doing practical support, washing sheets, or being in the homes of my friends and clients than what I noted as the "odor" of AIDS. Perhaps it was the ever-present complications of diarrhea or the drugs or the Kaposi's sarcoma lesions, but I think there is a distinct smell to the disease, at least for me. About four years ago, on the way to someone's home on the edge of the Tenderloin neighborhood in The City, I was walking down Taylor Street toward Sutter Street and stopped at a light with a group of people. There were a couple of obviously homeless men in front of me. I was very much in my head and not paying much attention to those around me when a breeze passed. They say that smell is one of the strongest memory triggers.

I literally felt a gut punch when a very distinctive and familiar odor came from one of the men in front of me. I had not experienced that odor in over 10 years but I knew exactly what it was. As I passed one of the gentlemen I glanced over and saw the Kaposi's sarcoma lesions on his face. It brought back the memory of all those men who had died and all that time spent trying to ease their passing. I know people passed me and wondered why I was weeping.

One of my dearest friends, Stevie, who was laughing and joking up until the very day he died from AIDS loved to quote a line from *The Wizard of Oz*. Always, after some amazing incident or goof up or embarrassing situation, Stevie would turn to me and laughingly say, "What did you learn, Dorothy?" Now I ask myself that question constantly about AIDS and the death of so many people dear to me and so many I only knew briefly. I never find the same answer. What did you learn, Dorothy? What indeed?

Once a Garden, Now a Wildflower

CARMEN MORRIS

EVERYONE HAS AT LEAST ONE thing they look forward to in their life. Whether it's sleeping in, making it to the weekend, finding their first love, or eating the last slice of chocolate cake waiting for them after a long, exhausting day. For me, however, the one most important thing of all I look forward to is making it through another day, happy and healthy. Many people look forward to waking up happy and healthy, but anyone who does is in a different book than mine. The chapters in my story are very long, with some pages straight and clean, others slightly torn and turning a bit brown in the corners. But I don't let those pages define me, and this is why.

I don't remember much from my childhood, but the things I do remember were never explained to me as a child; not until later in my life. Through the ages of walking and talking, I didn't know why I made so many trips to a big hospital. I didn't know why they had to draw my blood every time I went. I didn't know why my nanny was strict on making sure that I woke up every morning (six o'clock on the dot!) to take one nasty liquid medicine and one tasty one. I didn't know why I had to take this one nasty and one tasty medicine *every day*. I didn't know why I was the only one taking it and not my nanny or papa. However, I did know what they said when I had asked them why I was taking these nasty and tasty medicines. "It's to keep you healthy and alive," they had said. But wasn't I already healthy? And alive?

When you're a child, grownups don't tell you things. You think they do, but they don't. They really don't. And if they *do* tell you, then either they lie, exaggerate the truth, or don't tell you everything. I wasn't told everything.

When I said I don't remember much from my childhood, one of the things at the top of the list is my mom. As a child, I didn't remember much about her, and was told that she wasn't alive. My grandma told me before that I had attended her funeral when I was about four years old, but I don't remember it. When I had asked my nanny how my mother died, she just replied, "She didn't take her medicine that's supposed to keep her healthy. That's why it's super important that you take yours every morning, alright?" "Alright," I promised her.

The first time I heard the word HIV was in my last year of elementary school. That year, my grandma had finally told me that I had HIV, and I had no idea on earth what it was. In a short summary, she explained a few things to me that she said needed to stay between us and that they were very important in helping to protect not only myself, but others around me, including my friends. I wasn't allowed to share the same needle with anyone and I had to be extremely careful not to get my blood on anyone, especially if they had a cut or open sore on their body. (Because of my age at the time, my grandma didn't mention that bodily fluids were another way to spread the virus.)

Easy, I thought, until one day during recess I fell on the concrete and badly scraped my knee. A few of my friends around me were seconds from calling out for the teachers, but I refused the help. Confused, my friends all looked at me, one asking why I didn't want the teachers coming over. "Because I have HIV," I had told them. In the back of my mind, I was protecting my friends and the teachers. However, one teacher ended up noticing my accident and helped me to the nurse's office, away from my friends.

The following day, the same friend who asked why I didn't want help kept a bit of distance between the two of us the first half of the day until recess. I asked her if she was okay and she gave me a silent nod, but then said she couldn't talk to me. Shocked and slightly puzzled, I asked her why not and she said because she told her mom what happened yesterday at recess. More puzzled now, I asked her why doesn't her mom want her talking to me anymore? She replied, "She told me that because you have HIV, I can get it if I'm around you, so she told me not to talk to you anymore."

At that moment, I remember my skin getting hot because our group of friends had begun to crowd around us during the conversation. I remember feeling embarrassed, but I shook my head at her and said, "My grandma said I just can't share needles with anyone or get my blood on anyone's cuts." But this time she shook her head at me, saying "My mom told me I can't be around you because there's more of a chance that I will get it." We argued for a few minutes until my friend ended up saying that we can't be friends anymore.

That night I cried in my grandma's arms after telling her what happened. Grandma comforted me: "Her and her momma don't know a thing about you. If she doesn't accept you for who you are then she's not your true friend. Do you believe me?" I said, "I believe you." And I did. I truly did.

I didn't speak much about having HIV when I started middle school, except when I told my best friend and it made me feel closer to her because she didn't look at me as just someone who has HIV. I hated those weeks in health class though when they talked about diseases. I felt as if everyone knew I had HIV. Once I started high school, I told another one of my friends who I'd grown closer to in middle school. Again, it felt like a great weight had been lifted off my shoulders and I had nothing to hide. Then sometime in my junior year of high school a rumor started going around the school that I had AIDS. I didn't know how the rumor got started and I was too humiliated to get to the bottom of it. Soon I ended up just ignoring it until people stopped talking about it. At the time, I thought it was one of the worst things I could have experienced while living with HIV, but that was just the beginning.

A few months after I turned 17, I started working at the Food Lion grocery store. When summertime arrived, a lot of people came in for job interviews, but very few were hired. One of the new hires was a boy my age, but just a grade below me. He had blue eyes and his family came from the UK. We had kicked it off quite well in the first few months with a bit of flirtatious jokes while our coworkers teased us about being a couple. We showed a lot of interest in each other for a few months until we started dating. I didn't think we would get serious so quickly, so I didn't disclose my status with him as soon as we made it official. Some nights, we would get a bit intimate, but I stopped it before it could go any further than it should have.

After a few weeks, I realized my mistake of not telling him my status earlier and that I needed to do it now. I had felt this sick feeling in my stomach for a while now, almost like you've accidentally killed someone and now it was time to turn yourself in. I was at the point where I felt so guilty and selfish for not disclosing this to him sooner that when I finally did tell him, I didn't even care enough to think that I shouldn't talk to him about this at work. All hell broke loose at that point. Thinking about it today, it's all such a blur.

I remember bits and pieces of what happened, but I try not to remember because I'd never been so anxious and scared in my life. I just remember him shouting at me and pushing me away from him. He wouldn't even let me explain anything to him. He just heard the word "HIV" and started going mad. He said he needed space, and I gave it to him. For a few weeks I fell into a very weak and fragile state. This was someone that I had started to care a lot about who I lost, just like that. I started to overthink a lot of things, play a lot of different scenarios in my head about just what would have happened if I had told him straight up.

Every day for three months I had to speak to a counselor because I was unable to make it through the day without crying. I had harmed myself a few times because I felt absolutely disgusted with living with this. I thought to myself that no one wants to date or be in a relationship with someone who is living with HIV.

Only a few people knew about what happened with this incident, even though everyone at my job saw it take place. My two best friends, my family, my counselor, and my boss knew everything that happened. I'm very lucky to be close with my boss, because he became one of the very few people that I talked to everyday when everything was still happening. He gave me really good advice and was there to support me until I got better, and even to this day he's still always looking out for me.

Because of this horrible incident, I found an outlet in writing. Instead of bottling up all my feelings inside, I write them out as words on paper. So the good that came out of this would definitely be creating art with my experience. Anyone who is living with HIV/AIDS shouldn't let it define them as a person. You define it.

Now, I'm 19 years old, and a very happy 19-year-old at that. I've moved into my first apartment with my best friend of 15 years. So I'm finally taking that first real step into adulthood, and it's definitely scary. Oftentimes I have flashbacks to the first guy I fell in love with and how he broke my heart. Because of this experience, though, I believe that I grew stronger, both inside and out. I compare the experience to watching a wildflower grow back strong and healthy after being destroyed in a garden, because that's what I did. He and I once grew this garden together, but in the end, I became the wildflower.

Personal Turning Points

Baltimore's HERO

JACK B. STEIN

I WAS ANXIOUS AND EXCITED. It was 2008 and it had been a while since I'd been back in Baltimore. The Engineer's Club in the historic Mount Vernon district was an elegant and fitting setting for the 25th Anniversary Gala for the Health Education Resource Organization, known to everyone as HERO, Maryland's oldest and largest community-based AIDS service organization. In its early days, HERO was located in a medical arts building only a few blocks away and that is where I spent four years that changed my personal and professional life forever. AIDS did that to people.

In 1984 I moved to Baltimore to take a position as an entry-level therapist at a community mental health center just north of the city. I had recently completed my master's degree in social work from New York University (NYU) and was excited about this new venture.

While living in New York, I was among the first team of volunteer "crisis intervention counselors" with the Gay Men's Health Crisis (GMHC). At the time, GMHC was just getting established and still operating out of a modest four-story brownstone in Chelsea. Crisis intervention counselors were the first contact with someone requesting GMHC's services.

While a GMHC volunteer, I tried to do at least one or two intakes a week. GMHC was literally a lifeline for medical care and social services, or simply an outlet to talk with someone. AIDS was still a relatively new phenomenon in New York, and fear and stigma were rampant, fueled by prejudice and lack of understanding about how the virus was transmitted. Many of these intake interviews were held in cramped hospital rooms where I was required to wear a surgical gown, gloves, and a mask. During those early days, I harbored plenty of concerns about transmission and more than once I guiltily threw away the pen used to get a consent signature.

Upon arriving in Baltimore and seeing an advertisement in a local paper for volunteers, I placed a call to an organization called HERO. A few hours later, I found myself sitting in a small office speaking with the executive director, also a social worker. HERO had been founded the year before by a group of concerned Baltimore residents led by a local physician with a large and growing patient population affected by AIDS. The organization consisted mainly of a volunteer-based network offering a local AIDS hotline, a support group, advocacy services, and public education and outreach. By the time I left the meeting, somehow I had agreed to lead the weekly AIDS support group held in the home of a local volunteer.

My first support group meeting went nothing like I expected. About 15 men showed up. Only one man said he had AIDS, which was apparent from the many Kaposi's sarcoma lesions on his face and limbs. The rest of the men said they were HERO volunteer "buddies" and were there to provide support. It quickly became clear what was going on. Unlike New York, San Francisco, and Los Angeles, the number of people diagnosed with AIDS in Baltimore was still relatively low. Viral antibody testing was not yet available; consequently, the principal way one learned they were infected was when symptoms emerged. With the help of another volunteer who had counseling experience, we restructured the group to address the concerns of not only those with AIDS but the many more individuals who were uncertain of their health status, the so-called "worried well."

The following months were somewhat of a blur. More and more people began to be diagnosed and become ill. Community resources and skilled providers were still limited. I had already cut back my hours at the community mental health center to work part time at HERO, supported by a small grant from the Maryland Department of Health and Mental Hygiene. When eventually asked if I'd consider working full time at HERO, I paused only for a split second before I agreed. Few people were working in the AIDS field at the time and I had no idea what impact it would have on my professional career. I didn't care.

As HERO's first case manager, I was not at all prepared for the fact that many of our most needy clients also had substance use disorders. Baltimore had (and still has) a significant heroin problem, and with injection use as the major mode of administration, AIDS was not far behind. Unfortunately, I knew nothing about drug addiction or its treatment. I had received no formal training about substance use while getting my social work degree, and if a substance use disorder was detected on admission to the community mental health center where I first worked, the client would simply be referred to the addiction program down the hall, never to be seen again.

In those days (and still somewhat today), addiction was often ignored, denied, or marginalized. But HERO was different. We adhered to a philosophy that "AIDS does not discriminate" and were committed to serving anyone at risk for or affected by it. If it were not for the collaborative and giving spirit of the tight-knit group of local addiction treatment providers, many in recovery themselves, I'm not sure how we would have adequately served HERO's early clients.

Word of our efforts serving people who used drugs started to spread. In 1987, researchers from the University of Illinois at Chicago invited us to participate in a study funded by the National Institute on Drug Abuse to determine the effectiveness of an HIV prevention intervention using local peer outreach workers. Coupled with funds from the Baltimore City Health Department, we developed the Street Outreach AIDS Prevention Program (SOAPP), which consisted of a team of street-smart recovering drug users who had a level of dedication to AIDS prevention rivaled only by what I had observed in the gay community.

Watching the SOAPP team in action was something to behold. These men and women would work both day and night shifts canvassing some of the toughest neighborhoods in Baltimore and talking with anyone who would listen while they distributed literature, gave out free condoms, and demonstrated how to properly clean drug injection equipment with bleach. Occasional altercations with local police who would misperceive the outreach team's intentions resulted in the need to engage the Baltimore City Police Department in a partnership brokered by the Baltimore City Health Department. Eventually, it was decided to issue special identification cards to the SOAPP team verifying their role as community health outreach workers, which they would present to law enforcement officials if ever confronted.

During those early years, educational materials were at a premium nationwide and few AIDS service organizations or local health departments had the creative know-how and financial resources to generate their own informational sources for public dissemination. Through the efforts of a creative and entrepreneurial staff and a team of volunteers recruited from local advertising agencies, HERO developed a fund-generating publishing house to fill requests globally for an array of award-winning educational pamphlets, posters, training videos, and public service announcements. Orders literally began to pour in from all over the country and internationally for printed copies of our materials, which were often adapted to reflect local needs and services. The materials were often blunt and graphic, sometimes generating concern and objections from community members, especially when public funds were used to develop them. A favorite among the cutting-edge products was a series of condom "matchbook" covers with catchy phrases such as "An Ounce of Prevention," "Have a Lifesaver," and "A Ring for Your Next Engagement."

Like many AIDS service organizations during this time, HERO grew very rapidly in a short period. What had started as a small volunteer-based organization quickly morphed into a statewide agency with nearly 40 staff members and an annual budget over $1 million. And with that expansion came significant growing pains. Few of us had any real experience in managing a nonprofit organization and it began to show.

Differences of opinions regarding HERO's mission and priorities started to emerge among staff, the Board of Directors, and community advocates. Criticism was sharp at times. Questions arose regarding our level of dedication to the gay community, to what degree we should be focusing on education versus direct services, and whether we could adequately address the needs of minority populations. In response, other organizations began to pop up and eventually compete for limited funds once solely directed to HERO. Even larger, well-established organizations, such as the local chapter of the American Red Cross, began to compete for state grants to operate the AIDS hotline HERO had started years ago.

At one point, the sudden departure of a relatively new executive director over differences of opinion left HERO literally leaderless until I was eventually appointed director, a position I held for about a year and half until things began to stabilize. To help do so, we invited the Centers for Disease Control (before the agency added "Prevention" to its name) to conduct a program review of the organization and offer recommendations to the board of directors. The review was conducted over a three-day period in March 1988 by two CDC public health advisors who interviewed nearly 30 individuals from among HERO's staff, board of directors, funders, and major stakeholders. Their report included a number of helpful suggestions related to our mission and focus, organization and personnel management, program planning and evaluation, and fund raising strategies. The board of directors carefully reviewed the report and began work on addressing the findings and recommendations.

The CDC report was an important milestone for me personally. In addition to some very flattering words regarding my efforts to improve the organization's image, it noted that I was "overburdened" in my responsibilities. I suspect I was not alone in this regard as most AIDS service organizations were experiencing similar challenges in meeting the high demand for services with limited resources. In general, most staff were overworked and underpaid. Burnout was commonplace among AIDS service workers, and I was among those experiencing it. It became apparent to me that it was time to begin my transition from the organization. All of my predecessors left under less than ideal circumstances and I was determined not to repeat that trend. So, in summer 1988, I announced my departure to the board, providing what I hoped was ample time to plan a smooth transition into its next phase of leadership.

My four years in Baltimore had flown by in a heartbeat. During that time I had gained a lifetime of experience both personally and professionally. Never in my wildest dreams would I have envisioned this career path after graduating as a clinical social worker from NYU. And without my experiences at HERO I never would have made the leap to my subsequent professional experiences working at a national level on AIDS and substance use disorders.

Sitting in the audience at HERO's 25th Anniversary Gala 20 years later was bittersweet. By that time, I was a seasoned government employee, having made the transition to the federal workforce in 1997 that included a position in the Obama Administration's Office of National Drug Control Policy and my current position with the National Institute on Drug Abuse at the National Institutes of Health. Only a few of my colleagues from the early days were present at the gala. Most had moved on to new careers in different parts of the country. A few had succumbed to AIDS. I thought about the many clients and volunteers we had lost during that period before AIDS became a chronic but manageable condition.

Sadly, HERO closed its doors not too long after the gala. The newspapers reported the closure was due to financial mismanagement. I had heard rumors of those concerns for years but never got the full story. Perhaps I didn't really want to know the details. Despite the varied and interesting jobs I've held since then, my HERO days remain among my peak professional years. It was a time of creativity, growth, and innovation during an era of uncertainty, fear, and stigma. What better place for a young and idealistic social worker to have been? Looking back, there is so much for all of us who contributed to HERO to be proud of. For many of us, our early experiences with AIDS literally changed everything. AIDS did that to people.

But You're Not Part of Our Community

SUSAN M. KEGELES

IN MY LAST YEAR OF graduate school at the University of California, Berkeley, in 1984, I was a bit bored with my dissertation topic: how (heterosexual) couples made decisions about how many children to have. I knew that I wanted to blend social psychology with health issues, particularly reproductive rights issues or adolescent risk-taking behavior, but I wanted to do something more immediate and in line with my social justice orientation. I had engaged in anti–Vietnam War efforts, attending protests and organizing walkouts in high school and college, and I wanted my work to have a political, activist bent. But I didn't know how.

Every Sunday night when we'd get together, my brother Bob, who was a gay rights activist, would ardently educate me about the issues, including how sexual freedom is tied into human rights issues. He would regale me with anecdotes about the meaning of different colored handkerchiefs in gay men's back pockets; what slings at some bars were; what cruising was and where and how it was done; and what were common and more esoteric sexual practices among gay men. I knew this was meant to both educate and shock, so I became unshockable.

Bob and I were both proud that his activism, along with that of his colleagues, resulted in Berkeley being the first place in the United States to approve domestic partnerships. As much as I admired his activism, I didn't want to stop being an academic. I had worked hard for my PhD and wanted to use it. Besides, since childhood I had been fascinated by epidemics, specifically how humans made sense of the spread of fatal diseases, how they sought to avoid them, how they treat people who have them, and social and behavioral responses to them. But I was taught in graduate school that social and behavioral issues only pertained to chronic diseases, not to infectious diseases.

Bob was helping to run the Gay Men's Health Collective at the Berkeley Free Clinic. His role mostly consisted of giving injections or pills to men who had STIs (sexually transmitted infections). It was a good place, my brother thought, to meet like-minded men like himself, who had acquired a little curable infection now and then in their pursuit of fun with men. It was no big thing, until suddenly it was a huge thing.

Bob read the first *Morbidity and Mortality Weekly Report* from the Centers for Disease Control about an outbreak of something among gay men. Men began showing up at the Free Clinic for STI treatment who had something seriously wrong with them, such as generalized lymphadenopathy (abnormal enlargement of the lymph nodes) and were really sick. Over time, he realized something serious was going on and he shared his concerns with me about a disease called GRID (gay-related immune deficiency). At the time, epidemiological studies emerged showing that gay men who had multiple sex partners were getting sick.

Given that Bob had long since lost count of how many partners he'd had, we began to suspect that he might be at high risk for GRID. And I began to wonder how I might apply my social psychology and experimental research expertise to this new disease. As I started my first job at the University of California, San Francisco (UCSF), which focused on adolescent sexual and other risk behavior, there was a dispute in the field about the new test for HTLV-III, what GRID had begun to be called. What a person could do with the test result was confusing because it was not clear what caused the disease nor what someone could do to avoid contracting it. It was becoming pretty clear, however, that the disease had some connection with sexual activity, such as the use of "poppers" (amyl nitrate) with sex, the number of sex partners, contracting multiple STIs over time, and certain sex practices. Thankfully, it became clear that my dear, very sexually active brother might escape getting HIV since his sexual proclivities did not include anal sex.

I expressed my interest in working on this disease to my father (who was also a social psychologist working in public health), who coincidentally was on a conference panel with Tom Coates, a UCSF professor who spoke about the emergence of this new disease. Tom, upon hearing of my interests, told my father to have me meet with him, which I did. Tom's response when I met him was, "If you want to work in this field, write a grant proposal!" So I did, a very small one, and began collecting data at a newly opened "Alternative Test Site" where people in Oakland obtained HIV tests anonymously.

This led to a much larger study of Alternative Test Sites, including who obtained testing, what they did sexually, and what they planned to do with the knowledge of their HIV status. I began distributing surveys at Alternative Test Sites before and after testing. And I began to have my first experiences of a phenomenon I was to encounter frequently in my work: discomfort as a woman working with a population about which she might know little, in this case mostly white gay men. As I came to call it, the "Who Are You to Be Doing This Research?" question.

In my data collection, the Health Department had been greatly concerned that if heterosexual people seeking testing were exposed to the explicit sexual questions that I was asking of gay men, the straight people might be horrified. So I was required to seal the questions separately for gay men and straight people so that they had to break the seal to see the questions. At one test site, a gay man and his friend accidentally opened the "straight" seal and were a bit irritated (rightly so) about the questions because they were not focused on gay men's sexuality. When I referred them to the correct forms, they delighted in the questions and asked me, "How did such a *nice* girl learn about all these things?" I felt pleased, and vowed that I would work very hard to make sure that I could always present myself as extremely knowledgeable and informed when working with populations other than my own. It was clear that my credibility and the relevance of my work depended on it, both in my research methods and for outcomes.

Around this time, CAPS (the Center for AIDS Prevention Studies) came into existence. It was (and is) a research center that is grant funded by the National Institute for Mental Health. Suddenly, many of us were housed together, were networked, and had administrative staff. Up until this time, we were scattered around San Francisco because UCSF had no space for us. Ron Stall, Joe Catania, and I had shared an office over a Chinese restaurant. For meetings, we would cram together in a very small room at San Francisco General Hospital. All of a sudden we had a conference room that fit us all. Over time we got to know each other and developed a sense of community.

It seemed to me that nearly every man at CAPS was gay, and the women were 50:50 lesbian or straight. I didn't know everyone, but I loved the community. We were grateful to be working on AIDS prevention. Many of us were activists at heart as well as academics, wanting to put our research into the service of addressing social justice issues. We lost several colleagues: Leon McKusick, who was one of CAPS' "forefathers," and our business manager; Mark Gould; and Bobby Hilliard, one of the two men pictured on the cover of *Time* magazine about the "new gay movement," to name just a few. Many of my dear colleagues, especially those who were gay men, were losing their lovers and too many friends to AIDS.

Within a few years, I found Robert (Bob) Hays, a gay man who became my "*other* partner in life" (I already had a wonderful husband, Jeff Lazarus). One day, Tom Coates handed me a foot-high pile of applications for a postdoctoral position and told me to choose someone to work with. It was daunting. But Bob's application stood out. Not only was he a well-trained and published community psychologist, he stated that he was gay and wanted to work on research concerning gay men and the gay community. I appreciated that he was out about his sexual orientation and I needed help conducting research on gay men. I knew I needed to work with a gay man in order to conduct research regarding gay men's sexuality. When I met Bob in person, his beauty, with his dark brown hair and eyes, stunned me. He was shy and soft-spoken, although over time I realized he was strong and resolute in his beliefs and had a brilliant mind. He didn't trust me when we began working together and he was unconvinced that a straight woman could work on issues facing gay men.

Together, Bob and I developed the Mpowerment Project, an HIV prevention intervention for young gay men.[1] Our fields of training and life experiences complemented each other's, and I was determined to learn about gay men's sexual and social lives so that I could be a better researcher. Over time, Bob came to trust me. I knew this when he handed me a plain-looking European shampoo bottle with a label that said "Thanks for doing the do with me!" This was a reminder of working together in our first study community when a young man told us that the program we were developing should be as cool as a European shampoo bottle and used this phrasing to indicate working together. Faded as it is now, I continue to treasure it.

We continued testing Mpowerment in two consecutive projects, with young gay male communities in Santa Cruz and Santa Barbara, California, and Eugene, Oregon; and then tested it in Albuquerque, New Mexico, and Austin, Texas.[2] As Bob's health declined, we brought Greg Rebchook onto our team, another out gay man, who had both a PhD and considerable real-world experience in working at community-based organizations and health departments, deep compassion for others, and seemingly endless optimism. We continue to work together to this day. Mpowerment is now an intervention that has been implemented by more than 300 community-based organizations in the United States, and it is now being tested in Peru, South Africa, and Lebanon. As an HIV prevention intervention that focuses on empowerment, self-acceptance of being gay, community building, and critical consciousness, it goes beyond "simple" HIV prevention. Countless young men have expressed gratitude to me over the years for the development of Mpowerment, reporting that it changed their lives. To this day, I always talk of Bob and I as being codevelopers of the Mpowerment program.

The years of developing and testing Mpowerment were compelling, fascinating, tragic, productive, and reproductive for me. I delivered my first child, Paul, and went on maternity leave while Bob headed up data collection on our cohort of young gay men study. For several years Bob hid from me that he was HIV positive. He finally told me the truth the very day that I learned I was pregnant with my daughter, Rebecca, four years before discovery of antiretroviral medications was announced, which changed the course of the epidemic. I realized that Bob would die from AIDS at the same time I learned that new life was starting within me. He told me he had been diagnosed with AIDS the day I came home from the hospital having given birth to Rebecca. He died the day I was on a field trip with her fourth-grade class. The children, other parents, and teachers had gone to their bunks, and I stood at the pay telephone booth miles away from anything else and sobbed. I knew that I would need to go on with my life without my "other" life partner, but it was hard and felt so wrong. My life was rich with the daily activities of parenting children, while Bob and other gay men continued dying from AIDS. This dichotomy of dealing with life and death simultaneously served to deepen my commitment to fight AIDS among gay men. I wanted young gay men to live and flourish, as my own children were able to do.

Bob and I had decided the next two directions our research would take us, had he survived longer: adapting Mpowerment for young black gay men—the group at highest risk for HIV in the United States—and helping organizations implement the program effectively so that they could save lives. We thought that each of us would take one direction and support each other on the other direction. Instead, with Greg, I have pursued both.

I continue to address how a straight white woman can work with populations of which I am not a part. I learned the need to adopt an orientation of "cultural humility" with any new population. I know that I must listen and learn from those who are part of the group I am trying to reach and to be humble about my understanding of what it is like to live in a certain context with a sexual orientation different than mine. Many wonderful men have taught me about being a black gay man in this country, including John Peterson, Robert Williams, Venton Jones, Percy Rhodes, Greg Millett, Daryl Wheeler, Roosevelt Mosby, Hyman Scott, Sammy Nesbit, Terrance Anderson, Will Vincent, Michael Foster, Richard Hamilton, Bill Stewart, Haqumai Waring Sharpe, and Doran Senat.

Now my research on the Mpowerment Project extends to Peruvian, South African, and Lebanese young gay men, and hopefully, to young gay Thai men as well. I am inestimably grateful to my teachers, all of these men and many more, who taught me about their lives and trusted me to get to a place of understanding them and their communities.

References

1. Kegeles SM, Hays RB, Coates TJ. The Mpowerment Project: a community-level HIV prevention intervention for young gay men. Am J Public Health. 1996;86(8):1129–36.
2. Hays RB, Rebchook GM, Kegeles SM. The Mpowerment Project: community-building with young gay and bisexual men to prevent HIV1. Am J Community Psychol. 2003;31(34):301–12.

The Accidental Ethnographer

WILLIAM A. ZULE

The Intern

I had reservations about working with psychiatrists, but I had already quit my job and passed the point of no return. An hour before I arrived for my interview, they had received their official notice of grant award from the National Institute on Drug Abuse (NIDA) for the San Antonio National AIDS Demonstration Research (NADR) project. The NADR program was NIDA's first big foray into HIV prevention. David Desmond interviewed me, and toward the end of the interview he asked me if I knew anything about drugs. I reluctantly admitted that I knew quite a bit about them. I was a teenager in Austin, Texas, in the late 1960s and early 1970s, and drugs were everywhere. In 1968, I had worked as the janitor at the Vulcan Gas Company, Austin's original venue for psychedelic music and a haven for all kinds of drug users. Much to my surprise and relief, he told me that was great. David initially assigned me to search the case files from the 250 participants in the career study for reports of time that they had spent in methadone maintenance treatment and to code drug use, arrests, and employment status before, during, and after treatment.

A month into my internship, David asked me to conduct a literature review to determine when and why people who injected drugs switched from subcutaneous to intravenous injections. That turned out to be a challenging assignment, but I learned a great deal from the experience. My undergraduate studies did not prepare me to conduct a comprehensive literature review. In fall 1988, PCs still used DOS operating systems, online journals did not exist, and the computerized searchable databases at university libraries included very few journals.

I searched volumes of *Index Medicus* and the *Science Citation Index* by hand for articles. Each time after I read a relevant article or book, I reviewed the references and tracked down those that looked promising. By the end of the process, which took several months, I knew how to conduct a literature search. I had read numerous articles and books written from the mid-1800s through the 1960s. The information I gleaned about the history of needles and syringes, the history of injection, the history of needle sharing, and the origins and evolution of drug policy in the United States profoundly influenced my subsequent research and public health career.

In early November 1988, Ken Votsberger and David Desmond began interviewing and hiring staff for their new NADR project. They were interviewing candidates for various positions on the project, including outreach workers. I thought I could be an outreach worker, so I told David I was interested in applying for a position. He told me that he had another position in mind for me. He wanted me to be their ethnographer. I had no idea what an ethnographer was or what ethnographers do. Over the next few months I read a couple books on ethnographic methods[1,2] and several classic drug ethnographies, including "Taking Care of Business—The Heroin User's Life on the Street,"[3] *Ripping and Running,*[4] and *Wheeling and Dealing.*[5]

I completed my BA in December 1988. By the time David and Ken posted the ethnographer position in January of 1989, I had a fairly good idea of what ethnographers do, but I still needed to learn how to do it. Right after they posted the job, David sent me over to the University of Texas, San Antonio (UTSA), Office of Human Resources to apply. After some delays, they hired me as an ethnographer in March 1989. The leap of faith that led me to quit my job and attend school full time had resulted in a job that required a college degree. Of course it only paid $15,000 a year, which was less than most printing press operators made at the time.

The Rookie Ethnographer

With David's help I developed a semistructured interview guide that included topics Ken and David thought would be useful, plus a few of my own. Now I needed to find someone to interview. An urban ethnographer studying injecting practices among people who inject heroin, cocaine, and methamphetamine needs entrée into the local drug scene. Simply approaching people on the street and asking them if they inject illegal drugs can be counterproductive and potentially dangerous.

However, the local detoxification center allowed me to conduct interviews with their patients. I introduced myself to everyone in the dayroom and explained that I needed to interview people who inject drugs. A young woman agreed to let me interview her, and I interviewed 12 more people there over 2 weeks. After that I started going out with the outreach workers. Once people got used to seeing me with the outreach workers, I began conducting interviews on the streets. Initially I jotted down notes during the interviews and filled in the details between interviews. After the first 40 interviews, we decided to start tape recording them.

Pretty soon I started going out on my own and revisiting people I met through the outreach workers. On weekends, on my own time and using my own money, I would buy chicken, beer, and watermelon and hang out and grill with the people I interviewed. I ate with them, watched them prepare and inject their drugs, and observed their day-to-day activities and interactions. Later, I helped one of them enter treatment and get a job as an outreach worker for the project. He did well for several years before relapsing on heroin.

I liked doing research and decided to pursue a master's degree in sociology, so I went back to UTSA to discuss it with my undergraduate advisor. He asked me if I was more interested in theory or applied research. I told him that I was more interested in applied research. He suggested a degree in public health, which I never knew existed. He explained that the University of Texas School of Public Health (UTSPH) in Houston had a satellite campus in San Antonio that offered a master's in public health (MPH). I decided to go for it, took the Graduate Record Examination (GRE) in spring 1989, and started MPH classes in fall 1989.

The Crossroads of Ethnography and Public Health

Ethnography is not a 9-to-5 job, so my hours were flexible, which enabled me to work full time and take two classes each semester. The MPH courses fit perfectly with my work. Courses in epidemiology, the natural history of disease, and health promotion opened up a whole new world and gave me insights into my ethnographic observations.

One of my first observations related to how the social context surrounding the preparation, division, and injection of drugs influences risk behaviors and potential strategies for reducing these risk behaviors. Steve Koester, an ethnographer in Denver, had studied these practices.[6] At the same time, Jean Paul Grund, an ethnographer in the Netherlands, coined the term "frontloading" for the process of dividing liquefied drug solutions.[7] He later labeled the wider range of behaviors involved in preparing and dividing liquefied drug solutions as "syringe-mediated drug sharing."[8] Their work inspired my first published paper.[9] It replicated their findings and provided additional information regarding the social context in which these behaviors occur, the practical motivations of people engaged in them, and pragmatic strategies for eliminating the risk. I had published a brief report in 1990 on this in *Research in Progress*,[10] a NIDA publication. I approached David and Ken in 1991 and told them I wanted to turn the brief report into a full paper. They encouraged me to write the paper. I wrote it and submitted it in fall 1991. When I was getting ready to submit it, Fred Maddux told me, "You have the *nerve of failure*." To my utter amazement, I received an acceptance letter from the journal a couple months later.

My work as an ethnographer led me to examine differences between people who prefer heroin and those who prefer methamphetamine. I turned that into my MPH thesis in 1991, and I have continued to study how those differences influence HIV risk. I also noticed that many people who inject drugs have no interest in entering substance abuse treatment or in discontinuing drug use. This led to a long-term interest in how readiness for substance abuse treatment may influence the impact of treatment as an HIV prevention strategy.

The Power of Observation

Of greatest importance to me was my observation that syringes with detachable needles retain visibly more fluid and blood with the plunger depressed than insulin syringes with permanently attached needles retain. By 1991, most people who injected drugs in San Antonio injected with insulin syringes. One day I was sitting in a car with one of our outreach workers who had relapsed on heroin. He was injecting with a tuberculin syringe with a detachable needle that he had stolen from the project. After he finished injecting and drawing blood back into the syringe and reinjecting several times, he swore, "I hate these syringes. You can't get all the dope out of them." In an ethnographic eureka moment, everything fell together in my mind and I concluded that syringe design may play an important role in determining the course of an HIV epidemic among people who inject drugs.

Combining my new knowledge regarding disease transmission with observations of the injection process, I concluded that standard (high dead-space) syringes, such as tuberculin syringes, may retain hundreds or thousands of times more blood after injection and rinsing than insulin syringes would retain. I hypothesized that this would be enough to substantially alter the probability of HIV transmission if they were shared, and that the predominant type of syringe used in a city could influence the course of an HIV epidemic among people who inject drugs in that city.

Turning Research Into Practice

I completed my DrPH from the UTSPH in Houston in 1996, and I have continued to conduct research and test hypotheses regarding the impact of syringe design on HIV epidemics globally among people who inject drugs. Based on my research and that of others, in 2012 the World Health Organization recommended that needle and syringe programs offer "low dead-space insulin syringes to their clients,[11] and in 2015 the US Centers for Disease Control and Prevention released a bulletin that warned about the additional risk associated with sharing syringes with detachable needles.[12]

From an accidental ethnographer to a global applied scientist, I'm still asking questions, many that circle back to my beginnings, and working to make change. When I applied for the internship program, I was just hoping to get a job. I never expected to find a career.

References

1. Spradley JP. The ethnographic interview. New York: Holt, Rinehart and Winston; 1979.

2. Spradley JP. Participant observation. New York: Holt, Rinehart and Winston; 1980.

3. Preble E, Casey JJ. Taking care of business—the heroin user's life on the street. Int J Addict. 1969;4(1):1–24.

4. Agar M. Ripping and running; a formal ethnography of urban heroin addicts. New York: Seminar Press; 1973.

5. Adler PA. Wheeling and dealing: an ethnography of an upper-level drug dealing and smuggling community. New York: Columbia University Press; 1985.

6. Koester S, Booth R, Wiebel W. The risk of HIV transmission from sharing water, drug mixing containers and cotton filters among intravenous drug users. Int J Drug Policy. 1991;1(6):3.

7. Grund J-PC, Kaplan CD, Adriaans NFP, Blanken P. Drug sharing and HIV transmission risks: the practice of "frontloading" in the Dutch injecting drug user population. J Psychoactive Drugs. 1991;23:1-10.

8. Grund JP, Friedman SR, Stern LS, Jose B, Neaigus A, Curtis R, Des Jarlais DC. Syringe-mediated drug sharing among injecting drug users: patterns, social context and implications for transmission of blood-borne pathogens. Soc Sci Med. 1996;42(5):691–703.

9. Zule WA. Risk and reciprocity: HIV and the injection drug user. J Psychoactive Drugs. 1992;24(3):243–9.

10. Zule WA, Vogtsberger KN, Desmond DP. Needle risk behavior in San Antonio: an ethnographic perspective. Research in Progress (NIDA). 1990:38–40. Bethesda, MD: NOVA Research.

11. World Health Organization. Guidance on prevention of viral hepatitis B and C among people who inject drugs. World Health Organization; 2012.

12. Centers for Disease Control and Prevention. Hepatitis C and injection drug use. Atlanta, GA: (US) Centers for Disease Control and Prevention; 2016. Retrieved May 1, 2017, from https://www.cdc.gov/hepatitis/hcv/pdfs/factsheet-pwid.pdf

People Who Use Drugs

GRID
Gay-Related Immune Deficiency

JAMES L. SORENSEN

I THINK THE YEAR MUST have been 1981. I was waiting to interview research participants at the methadone clinic at San Francisco General
Hospital (SFGH). We had just finished a study aiming to detoxify people
from heroin in 3 or 6 weeks, using either methadone or LAAM (levo-alpha-
acetylmethadol), a synthetic opioid that lasted longer than methadone and
was supposedly easier to "detox" from. We were starting to recruit patients
to get off of methadone at a therapeutic community, where the program was
friendly to people who wanted to detoxify from methadone. The head of the
therapeutic community was a former methadone patient. At the time, my
focus was finding ways to help people get off of drugs, including getting off
of methadone.

The first methadone program in San Francisco had opened a dozen years
before. The treatment was popular with injection drug users, and half a
dozen clinics had sprouted up in the city, supported by federal initiatives to
cut drug-related crime and increase employment. I had a picture of Supervisor Dianne Feinstein opening the Westside Methadone Clinic. By 1981, Supervisor Feinstein had become Mayor Feinstein, and later she would be the
long-time senator from California. As the treatment grew, methadone was
drawing increasing fire from the public, with headlines like "Once called a
solution, methadone is now a problem"[1] and "At methadone clinics, old
habits die hard."[2] There were political and ethical objections to providing
indefinitely long stints of methadone maintenance treatment.

I thought I was on my way to a career developing ways to get people off
of methadone maintenance safely and back into mainstream society, when
I spied a green flyer on the floor. I picked it up and saw it was old, somewhat torn, and photocopied from a handmade original. I was struck by the

biggest feature, a drawing of two men, one massaging the other's back. Neither one was wearing a shirt. "What is this?" I asked one of the nurses. The nurse explained to me, "They're calling it a gay plague. People are getting sick and don't know why. No one knows what the cause is." The flyer labeled it "GRID," for gay-related immune deficiency. The flyer had a brief explanation that people were coming down with rare cancers and an unusual kind of pneumonia, and their immune system was compromised. There was a meeting where you could learn what you could do to help, but by this time the date had already passed. Seeing that GRID flyer at the methadone clinic is my first memory about what would become acquired immunodeficiency syndrome.

GRID was only one of the names given to what eventually became known as AIDS. This was the case when I read the green flyer. Early reports in Los Angeles, New York, and San Francisco identified cases among gay men and looked for a common cause for the problem, identifying factors that included gay sexual practices, use of inhalant stimulants, and attendance at bathhouses where gay sexual activities occurred. Quickly, the early studies also identified other groups with the same problem, including injection drug users, babies born to addicted women, and recipients of blood products such as hemophiliacs. Eventually, it was clear that the problem was not limited to gay men, and the cause was related to a toxic agent borne by blood and "bodily fluids." On July 27, 1982, at a meeting with representatives from many interest groups in attendance, the Centers for Disease Control decided to label the problem as acquired immunodeficiency syndrome (AIDS).

It took some time after seeing the flyer, but my focus changed dramatically. In 1982, I began leading the San Francisco General Hospital drug abuse treatment program, and we focused more and more on AIDS. I remember presenting a poster about treating drug users with AIDS in our treatment program at the 1986 American Psychological Association convention.[3] Don Des Jarlais and I had the only posters about AIDS (placed adjacent to each other), and almost no one came up to talk with us. Over time, my efforts changed from trying to help people to get off of methadone to trying to get them on it and to stay on it so their HIV risk would be reduced. Methadone became a tool in the growing "harm reduction" approach.

New scientific and treatment partnerships emerged. I remember one time in the 1980s when Andrew Moss dropped by my office. Dr. Moss was an epidemiologist at the University of California, San Francisco and SFGH. He asked me whether people really stopped taking heroin when they got on methadone. I explained that urine testing showed many of them did, and clearly most reduced their heroin use dramatically. He did some calculations with me. I don't remember the details, but it was something like this: If there were 10,000 heroin users in the city, and the rate of HIV infection was 4 percent, if we could get all 400 on methadone we could stop the epidemic! This was in a time when methadone was under attack, and at SFGH we were fighting to keep the 150-patient clinic open. I was skeptical that (1) the city would provide any more methadone treatment "slots," (2) we could identify the 400 people, and (3) they would want to get on methadone treatment. The idea was a good one, but it seemed impractical. Looking back, I wish we had fought for that idea.

Our partial solution was to make having AIDS a priority for admission to the methadone program. Our first patients were a couple who lived in a single-room occupancy hotel. Neighbors had spray-painted "Go Away AIDS" on their door. Patients were clearly stigmatized, and people worried about the health of people treating these patients. Over time, the number of AIDS patients grew, and in partnership with the hospital's outpatient AIDS program the patients could get primary medical care at the methadone program. Despite the medical care, many patients perished. Initially, we held a memorial service when patients died, but over time there were so many that we held a service just twice yearly.

Over the years, we developed HIV/AIDS education programs for those in detoxification, methadone maintenance, and therapeutic communities, and we developed adherence intervention strategies to help people who inject drugs to take medications more reliably. These poignant memories of early times coping with HIV/AIDS among drug users were prefaced by finding a flyer about GRID.

References

1. Hillstrom T, Tulley AI. Once called the solution, methadone now a problem. The Palm Beach Post. 1974. p. 46.

2. Gregg SR. At methadone clinics, old habits die hard. The Washington Post. 1981 Jun 4; Sect. 1, 3.

3. Sorensen JL, Batki SL, Faltz B, Madover S. Treatment of AIDS in substance abuse programs. In: Meeting of the American Psychological Association. Washington, DC; 1986.

Stories and Lessons Learned Surrounding People Who Inject Drugs

The Early Days of the HIV/AIDS Epidemic

ROBERT E. BOOTH

I

N 1986, BEFORE THE ADVENT of e-mail or text messaging, Nick Kozel, head of the Community Epidemiology Work Group (CEWG) at the National Institute on Drug Abuse (NIDA), called me. CEWG, which was supported by NIDA, comprised local drug abuse experts who reported semiannually on drug trends in sentinel sites, including major metropolitan areas and states. The genesis for the CEWG was to provide a rapid assessment of drug trends to alert government and health officials of what may become problematic. It was designed to assess current and emerging drug abuse patterns, developments, and issues using multiple sources of information—such as emergency room admissions, overdose deaths, substance use treatment admissions, and drug price and purity. This unique epidemiology network functioned from 1976 to 2014, with the 76th and final CEWG meeting held in June 2014.

The CEWG provided a foundation for continuity in the monitoring and surveillance of drug problems and related health and social consequences, and it was among the first organizations to draw attention to designer drugs, crack cocaine, and HIV among people who inject drugs (PWID). As director of research and evaluation for the Colorado Alcohol and Drug Abuse Division, I served as the Denver representative to the CEWG from 1977 to 1986.

The purpose of Nick's call was to ask if I would be interested in interviewing newly admitted methadone maintenance patients who injected drugs as part of a multicity appraisal of HIV-related risk behaviors. Six to eight of us were recruited to conduct interviews, including John Watters in San Francisco and Wayne Wiebel in Chicago. We were asked to interview recent admissions, as they would recall their injecting behaviors since they were just off the street and because NIDA did not know if we could recruit out-of-treatment PWID from the streets. We aimed to interview 20 patients from methadone clinics, as well as other clinics if they treated PWID, located throughout the various target cities. Participants were paid $10 for their time and the clinic would receive $5 for the referral. An information sheet describing the project and its purpose was posted at the reception desk. Individuals agreeing to participate were asked to call the study investigator for that city. However, in one case I was offered an office at the clinic to wait for new admissions who, upon reading the information sheet, could come to me for the interview using a questionnaire developed by NIDA. In general, clinics were quite willing to be part of the study. In fact, one clinic director told me she was pleased to participate as the $10 stipend would help pay for the clients' methadone dose.

Stories Told and Lessons Learned

Story 1—A white female, approximately 30 years of age, had been injecting heroin for around ten years. She came from a very wealthy family and was considered, by her own admission, to be the "black sheep" of the family. I asked her if she used a new needle every time she injected. She said, "I may be a junkie but I'm not stupid, I don't want to die." Clearly, she was well informed about the risk of needle sharing.

Story 2—A Hispanic male in his mid-50s, a Rapid Transit bus driver, injected cocaine. He said he injected mainly on the weekends and that his wife, who did not inject, was usually home at the time. He had informed her not to report him or she would get in trouble because she was a coconspirator. In the interview, we asked people about injecting intravenously, skin popping, and injecting intramuscularly. Other than this individual, no one reported injecting intramuscularly. When asked about this, he replied that he always injected both intravenously and intramuscularly (in his buttocks) and at the same time. He said, "When the vein gives out, the ass kicks in."

Story 3—A well-dressed white woman in her late 30s, who could have passed as an executive, was a heroin injector. Because I could not imagine her on the streets copping dope, I asked how she obtained her drugs. She said from her boyfriend, who was a major dealer in Denver. I asked if he injected as well, to which she replied "no," as it was purely business.

Story 4—A Hispanic female in her early 20s who was a cocaine injector. I asked if she ever shared needles; she said "No, I never share." Later, I asked about injecting with various people in her life. She told me that she always injected with her aunt, that they would save up their money, buy all the cocaine they could afford, and spend the weekend injecting until it was gone. I mentioned that earlier she had told me that she never shared needles. She replied that she didn't share, that they purchased the drugs and needles/syringes together. Thus, they both owned them and did not share. This led later to a change in the NIDA questionnaire during the Cooperative Agreement, a large national study with 23 sites for HIV prevention. Instead of asking about needle sharing, participants were asked, "How many times (in the past 30 days) did you use a needle/syringe that you *know* had been used by someone else?"

. . .

Conclusion

These few examples of PWID point to the diversity and heterogeneity of this population, from street addicts to blue-collar to white-collar workers. Until the AIDS epidemic, there had been no large-scale studies of PWID, other than among persons incarcerated or in drug treatment facilities, typically residential treatment. A number of ethnographic and qualitative studies had been done, such as *Ripping and Running: A Formal Ethnography of Urban Heroin Addicts* by Michael Agar in 1973, but no large studies had been conducted of PWID who were not "captured" in one way or another. Consequently, numerous myths were prevalent concerning drug users: they cannot be located; they will not sit down to be interviewed about illicit and sensitive activities; they will not tell the truth; and they will not give accurate locator information and consequently cannot be followed over time. Countless investigations have subsequently revealed the falsity of these myths, including two large multisite studies, the National AIDS Demonstration Research (NADR) project and the Cooperative Agreement, both funded by NIDA.

We began our work in Denver in 1987 and have been in continuous operation ever since. Over the course of 30 years, we have recruited and intervened with thousands of PWID. We may, in fact, be one of the longest if not the longest running project in the world devoted to providing and evaluating interventions with PWID. They are indeed a diverse group, an important group in the substance-using culture that still deserves attention.

Encounter With the Dark Side

WAYNE WIEBEL

Setting the Stage

In transitioning from the early to mid-1980s, it became apparent that the shadow of the HIV/AIDS epidemic was rapidly spreading over Chicago. Any hope of somehow avoiding the well-documented experiences of San Francisco and New York were quickly vanishing. After all, the city had substantial subpopulations of men who had sex with men and injection drug users, and there was no reason to believe that the way they had sex or administered drugs was any different from other places where HIV outbreaks had occurred.

As a substance abuse epidemiologist for the Illinois Dangerous Drugs Commission, I was concerned about the new public health threat involving injection drug users. A Community Epidemiology Work Group meeting at the Centers for Disease Control, visits by Dr. Harold Ginsberg of the National Institute on Drug Abuse (NIDA), and a growing body of literature, including attention in the popular media, contributed to a growing recognition of what was already under way.

The state's single state authority (SSA) for drug treatment and prevention in Illinois needed to do something. Randall Webber, a street drug pharmacologist and head of prevention at the SSA, eagerly joined forces with me in developing a game plan. We received approval for the time and resources required to train drug treatment nurses in universal precautions as well as all drug treatment staff in what was known about the spread of HIV and how infection could be prevented. Curricula were drafted and trainings scheduled to be delivered by Randy and me in methadone and other treatments programs that included injection drug users among clients across Illinois.

It soon became clear that, while a worthwhile first step, the trainings were nowhere near sufficient to have much impact in limiting further spread of the infection. Counselors were encouraged to share what they were learning about preventive measures with clients but often expressed reservations about doing so—not so much in relation to safer sex and condom promotion, but the prospect of addressing needle-borne risk-reduction measures with clients in drug treatment often met with opposition. The counselors were well aware of the frequency of relapse among their clients, particularly methadone patients, as a consequence of regularly scheduled toxicology screens. Yet there seemed to be some sort of therapeutic barrier to the discussion of safer injection practices with clients in that it acknowledged the potential of relapse. Some counselors thought it best to withhold discussion until their clients did relapse, but that might well be too late.

Difficulties were likewise encountered in suggesting that clients share risk-reduction messages with friends who continued to inject drugs. Counselors wanted their clients to distance themselves from active users, not encourage engagement. Moreover, those in treatment represented but a small proportion of those at risk and arguably were already at decreased risk by virtue of being in treatment. Any hope for containing the epidemic would require something being done to address the much larger numbers of active injection drug users not in treatment.

Suggestions to reach out to active injection drug users in community settings were greeted with disinterest by the SSA. Their position was that the agency's responsibilities in the community did not extend beyond the four walls of the programs they funded. For the time being, progress was at a standstill.

Meanwhile, nascent outreach programs targeting injection drug users for the purpose of preventing further spread of HIV were getting under way in Baltimore and San Francisco. In Rockville, MD, George Beschner, who headed up the Community Research Branch at NIDA, was beginning to put in motion plans for what a few years later would become the National AIDS Demonstration Research project (NADR).

In Chicago, Norman Altman, a colleague who had done data analysis on a number of NIDA grants I worked on while at the University of Chicago, invited me to a series of informal meetings with gay activists concerned about mounting responses to the threat of AIDS. They, like Chet Kelly, the newly appointed official overseeing AIDS at the Chicago Department of Health, and Dr. Renslow Sherer from the Sable-Sherer AIDS Clinic at Cook

County Hospital, were all concerned about injection drug users but uncertain about what could be done. After all, many in the public health field reasoned that this hidden population would be difficult to reach, and even if engaged, would not likely embrace attempts to change their behavior. Addiction itself implied a loss of control, and addicts risked overdose death every time they injected. Yet the stage was set with a supporting cast of characters eager to listen, critique, and most of all encourage ideas about what might be done to contain further spread of HIV among injection drug users. Opportunity was ripe. Ideas for adapting the earlier work of Dr. Patrick Hughes[1] intervening in outbreaks of heroin addiction in South Side Chicago neighborhoods to address the challenge of HIV transmission among injection drug users became a preoccupation.

A Rude Awakening

On one otherwise uneventful day in 1985, I received a telephone call from a psychiatrist and prominent figure in the substance abuse treatment field who ran one of the largest methadone programs in Illinois. He knew that I was working on plans for an HIV/AIDS intervention targeting injection drug users and called me about a very troubling situation he had just learned about. Apparently, one of his patients from a community mental health center was a cleric entangled in a rescue mission involving a young heroin-addicted male prostitute. The young man had recently been diagnosed with AIDS and had become fixated on infecting as many fellow addicts as he could. The cleric became increasingly traumatized at his inability to convince the young addict to stop infecting others. As was the case with preventing HIV transmission among injection drug users in general, so it was in this instance as well. Something clearly needed to be done, but what should be done was not at all evident.

Sufficient time has passed that neither the psychiatrist nor I remember all the details of that telephone conversation some 30 years ago. However, we explored a number of potential game plans and agreed to collect additional information before resuming the conversation. The psychiatrist would find out all he could about what the young addict was doing to infect others and where he was doing it. I would explore two possible avenues of action—the first external, through the Department of Public Health; the second internal, through engaging the addict subculture.

Fortunately for me, the director of the Illinois Department of Public Health, Dr. Bernard Turnock, was an acquaintance whose office was not far from mine in the new State Office Building. A meeting was set up in short order and I shared what I knew with him. The option of quarantine was dismissed relatively quickly. Given the lack of evidence to substantiate the basic facts surrounding the case, not knowing the identity of the individual, and the need for a rapid response to halt further transmission, invoking this containment measure proved to be untenable.

That left the option of attempting an independent community-based intervention. As it so happened, plans already in the works for adapting Hughes' neighborhood heroin epidemic intervention model to address the HIV/AIDS epidemic among injection drug users offered more promise. The framework for what would become the Indigenous Leader Outreach Model (ILOM) was still only in its infancy. Yet the first three of what would become five objectives included in the ILOM intervention manual[2] were already appearing in early drafts of an intervention strategy: (1) to identify and gain access to individuals at risk; (2) to increase awareness of HIV and how it is transmitted; and (3) to promote a range of viable risk-reduction strategies. What was not yet clear was how to move from strategy to action plan.

My next conversation with the psychiatrist underscored the urgency of the situation. Despite his patient's pleas with the young addict to cease intentionally infecting others, the young man showed no remorse or interest in curtailing his dangerous behavior. To the extent he was successful in transmitting HIV, in those days prior to the advent of antiretroviral therapy, it was evident to all of us that the disturbed youth's actions were pretty much synonymous with handing out death sentences.

In following up with his patient, the psychiatrist was able to collect details relating to the patterns of behavior the young addict revealed to the cleric. He would frequent shooting galleries on the West Side of Chicago and share syringes with anyone inclined and/or in need of doing so. Late in the evening the young man would phone the cleric and ask to be picked up. Increasingly desperate appeals to cease intentionally infecting others fell on deaf ears, and the cleric grew more distraught at his inability to influence his wayward acquaintance. The cleric was not ready to reveal the identity of the youth but did agree to provide the names of the street intersections where he had picked him up after being called to the rescue. Exactly where the shooting galleries were located was not known, but fortunately I knew someone who probably did, Armando Lira. Armando was a veteran who got addicted to heroin in Vietnam and was struggling to free himself from dependence when I met him about seven years previously. As a Marine veteran, he was both tough as nails and skillful in his ability to secure the attention of others. At the same time, he was a man of heartfelt concern and effervescent sincerity. When Armando spoke, people listened.

A Game Plan Unfolds

Armando retained close ties to the injection drug user subculture on Chicago's West Side, where he was well known and held in high regard. On the streets, where treachery is common currency and friendships can be fleeting, Armando had the reputation of being trustworthy whenever he gave his word and someone who would not stand down if challenged. If anyone could gain access to neighborhood shooting galleries, convey credible alarm, and prompt preventive measures, Armando was our best bet.

I set up a meeting with Armando and briefed him on the situation. He grasped the gravity of the predicament in short order. Instead of a gun and bullet, our disturbed sociopath was using a syringe and virus. Instead of a loud report of gunfire bringing immediate consequences, our silent killer and his victims were operating in an opiate haze with fatal consequences not likely evident for years. Once again, clearly, something needed to be done. Armando enthusiastically agreed to help out and asked for the identity of the perpetrator. His solution was far simpler and quite likely more effective than my game plan. He would put word out on the street what this "murderer" was doing and street justice would most assuredly be swift. For a moment I was taken totally aback. Not so much as a consequence of feeling that this would be wrong but in recognizing that this option, that hadn't even occurred to me, was just so remarkably straightforward and efficient.

As his suggestion sunk in, I realized that it was probably very fortunate that I didn't know the identity of this young man. I sensed that I needed to impress upon Armando that we would unlikely be able to find out his identity even if we were to try. That opened the door to the plan B that I had been working out in my mind as the situation unfolded. Fortunately, Armando's enthusiasm to be of assistance did not waver.

Borrowing from the HIV prevention strategies I was working through as an intervention model targeting injection drug users, I laid out my game plan and its requirements to Armando. First, we would need to identify and gain access to those injection drug users who our perpetrator was targeting as victims. We knew the young addict was frequenting shooting galleries on the West Side, and we knew the nearby street intersections where the cleric would be asked to pick him up late at night. I inquired if Armando could find the shooting galleries near these street intersections and he assured me it wouldn't be a problem. Any that he wasn't already aware of, he could easily find out about through asking acquaintances. Next I wondered if Armando would be able to gain entry and talk to those present. Again, he told me that this would not be a problem. So far, so good.

Second, we needed to make sure occupants of the shooting galleries were aware about HIV/AIDS and familiar with how it can be transmitted through the sharing of injection paraphernalia. I explained to Armando that HIV spread like hepatitis when someone uses a syringe that had previously be used by someone else who was already infected. He got it straightaway and registered it together with his far more nuanced understanding of injection practices than I would ever possess. The challenge, I suggested, would be having him convey this to the injection drug users he encountered together with the alarming fact that someone unknown to us was getting high there and suspected to be intentionally infecting others through sharing syringes.

Finally, he would need to provide those he engaged with risk-reduction alternatives they could adopt to prevent further spread of infection. The first and most effective option would be to stop sharing syringes. This would be possible for some injection drug users some of the time, but we realized that universal compliance would be elusive. Although there was a vibrant black market in syringes, the law still required a prescription and anyone caught possessing a syringe without a prescription could be charged. Further, the use of a new, sterile syringe for each injection at this point in time was virtually unheard of outside of injection drug users in the medical professions. As a backup measure, I considered promoting bleach disinfection in instances where a new syringe was not available. Word had come that this was already being piloted in San Francisco with some success. Injection drug users there seemed receptive to flushing out previously used syringes with bleach when faced with the prospect of having to use one already used by someone else. Armando expressed willingness to bring bleach to the shooting galleries he would visit and explain its use as a preventive measure. Prospects for putting our plan into action seemed all clear. We set a date and time to meet up on the West Side to start the process.

I bought a carton of bleach, threw it in the back of my car, and picked up Armando as planned. Looking back on it now, I don't recall any hesitation or reservation. Perhaps we were just blindly unaware of all that might go wrong. What I do recall is a shared sense of importance about the task at hand and a commitment to see it through to the end.

We began by looking for parking places close to the street intersections provided by the patient. Any consideration of joining Armando in visiting the shooting galleries had been dismissed by the time we commenced. No advantage in attempting to do so was apparent. He alone would take a gallon bottle of bleach and disappear for 30 minutes to an hour. Upon return I would quiz him on how it went and each time he would assure me that it went well and that there were no problems. It was frustrating, I recall, having to sit alone imagining what was transpiring in the nearby shooting gallery (where one could buy drugs, rent shooting equipment and do their drugs). Once one intervention had concluded, Armando's focus shifted to the next place he was going. In this community area, most occupants would likely be Spanish speaking, but some individuals present might only speak English. Armando was on a mission, and there was not much time for conversation or discussion, in the shooting gallery or with me. Knowing him, I imagined he pleaded with occupants to listen as he had a very important message to deliver; demonstrated concern about their plight in explaining the situation; convincingly responded to questions about avoiding exposure; and then respectfully excused himself in needing to move on to the next gallery.

In hindsight, without direct observation and only limited feedback, it seems curious I was so pleased at the time with how things seemed to be going. Then again, there was not the least shadow of a doubt that Armando was incensed about the situation we were attempting to remedy and fully invested in preventing this guy from infecting anyone else. It took a few days to cover all the shooting galleries Armando was able to identify. Each day we debriefed and I was able to discover much more about what happened. Among the variable numbers of individuals encountered at the different galleries, there was much surprise, some denial, but mostly anger at what they were being told had happened without their knowledge. According to Armando, the combination of anger and concern he was able to generate left his audience very receptive to suggested risk-reduction measures. Unfortunately, we'll never know how many individuals embraced which risk-reduction alternatives for how long. I would guess that the rumor about someone intentionally infecting others through sharing syringes would have spread like wildfire through the injection drug user networks that frequented these galleries. We can only hope that once the perpetrator learned that his contemporaries were on the lookout for him, he stopped trying to infect others. At any rate, based on little more than impression, both Armando and I were about as pleased as could be with what had been accomplished.

The Aftermath

At the time, I don't recall thinking about what Armando did as demonstrating the potential of the Indigenous Leader Outreach Model intervention strategies I had begun to organize on paper and share with colleagues. Yet it must have bolstered my enthusiasm for the plans I was developing and added to confidence that I was on the right track. By 1986, CDC funds through the Chicago Department of Health were secured to formally launch a small-scale ILOM intervention pilot.

Then, in 1987, George Beschner's NADR initiative from NIDA came to fruition.[3] We were fortunate enough to be included among the first round of awardees and with the substantial resources available, scaled up seemingly overnight to establish community-based field stations on Chicago's North Side, West Side, and South Side.

Three ethnographers were tasked with supervising intervention and research operations out of the field stations: Wendell Johnson on the South Side, Lawrence Ouellet on the North Side, and Antonio Jimenez on the West Side. What they were able to accomplish with their teams of indigenous outreach workers in short order is nothing less than amazing. Any doubt about the ability to access this "hidden population" in community settings was quickly put to rest. First-round data, including completed questionnaires and serologic samples, were collected from 1,023 active injection drug users. Of these, the ethnographers were able to determine that 850 belonged to major injection drug user social networks from communities surrounding the field stations and would be followed in our longitudinal cohort study.[4]

By 1988, analysis of first-round NADR data collection in Chicago revealed unanticipated HIV seroprevalence results.[5] Already known was the fact that HIV was present among Chicago injection drug users based on diagnosed AIDS cases and HIV antibody testing of drug treatment entrants and samples from those incarcerated. Yet the prevalence rate among injection drug users in general and how it might vary across community areas was not known. The NADR sample showed 18 percent of injection drug users from the historic hub of the heroin scene on Chicago's South Side to be HIV infected. A suspected epicenter of infection caused by overlapping gay and injection drug user social networks on the North Side had a 23 percent prevalence rate. Finally, that the West Side topped infection rates with 34 percent testing positive came as a surprise.

The largely Puerto Rican population of injectors in this community may well have been exposed early on to HIV through relations in New York City and Puerto Rico. Additionally, looking back on the disturbing case of the intentional infector on Chicago's West Side raises the question of what, if any, influence that may have had in catapulting HIV prevalence there. Regrettably, one can only wonder.

References

1. Hughes P. Behind the wall of respect: community experiments in heroin addiction control. Chicago, IL: University of Chicago Press; 1977.

2. Wiebel WW. The indigenous leader outreach model: intervention manual. US Department of Health and Human Services. NIH Publication No. 93-3581. Rockville, MD: National Institutes of Health; 1993.

3. Brown BS, Beschner GM, editors. Handbook on risk of AIDS injection drug users and sexual partners. Westport, CT: Greenwood Press; 1993.

4. Wiebel WW, Jimenez A, Johnson W, Ouellet L, Jovanovic B, Lampinen T, et al. Risk behavior and HIV seroincidence among out-of-treatment injection drug users: a four-year prospective study. J Acquir Immune Defic Syndr Hum Retrovirol. 1996;12(3):282–9.

5. Wiebel WW. Combining ethnographic and epidemiologic methods in targeted AIDS interventions: the Chicago model. Rockville, MD: National Institute on Drug Abuse Research Monograph 80, DHHS Publication No. (ADM)88-1567; 1988.

Junkiebonden and Users' Groups

Learning About the Collective Organization
of People Who Use Drugs

SAMUEL R. FRIEDMAN

A T THE END OF 1983, after many months of unemployment, I got a job as a project director and researcher on Don Des Jarlais' (at that time, the deputy director of the Bureau of Research of the New York State Office of Drug Abuse Services) Risk Factors project that was trying to understand AIDS among people who injected drugs. I knew remarkably little about drug use or the people who used drugs, and even less about viruses, diseases, and related subjects. In some ways, my ignorance may have served me and public health well, as it meant I had fewer fixed preconceptions about these topics than people who had more experience. Though I had been exposed to the way the media and other cultural forms treated drug users, I knew enough from my years fighting racism and war that the content of such messages was likely to be inaccurate and biased. Consequently, although I had a lot to learn very fast, I was very open to it.

Within a year or so, after analyzing data we had collected that showed many similarities between the ways persons who inject drugs thought about and interacted about AIDS and the ways that gay men did,[1,2] I developed a hypothesis that many of my coworkers at the time thought was very strange—namely that in spite of the problems of addiction, stigma, and fear of arrest that people who inject drugs face, they could themselves set up organizations to fight the spread of HIV and to help the sick, much like gay men and their allies had done. A few months after developing this hypothesis and beginning to put together the analyses to show it, one of my colleagues, Herman Joseph, told me that he had been at a conference in Europe where the distinguished drug researcher Charlie Kaplan had told him that drug users in the Netherlands had organized *Junkiebonden*, or drug users' unions. Because I knew Dr. Kaplan from my years as a sociology professor at UCLA (where he was then a graduate student), I contacted him about this. We arranged a two-week trip for me to see how the users' unions functioned. Charlie let me stay in his apartment in Rotterdam (while he and his family were absent) and arranged for Wouter de Jong to introduce me to these groups and their activists. This started a collaboration and friendship with Wouter that led to many publications and a lasting friendship.[3,4]

During this and subsequent visits, I spent a lot of time at the Rotterdam *Junkiebond* and at other groups in Amsterdam, Groningen, Lelystad, Nijmegen, and elsewhere. This was the first time I had any lengthy interaction with drug users. It was quite easy for me because Wouter was well known and trusted by the members of the users' groups and because I had a long history of social activism myself. I learned that they had developed innovative HIV prevention methods and had also conducted effective campaigns for changes in Dutch policies and programs related to drug use and drug users. I was impressed by the fact that meetings of drug user activists I attended were conducted at least as well as university and college department meetings I had been part of—in spite of the fact that the chair of the drug users' meeting (and other participants) might be smoking heroin during the meeting. Similarly, I would often interview people about their activities while they were high and this would not interfere with our being able to have deep and meaningful conversations.

I also noticed that there were a number of different types of groups that went by the name *Junkiebond*.[3,5] The Rotterdam group had been started by friends who knew each other growing up in youth homes and, in some cases, from membership in radical political groups. They became drug users and learned firsthand the ways police and treatment authorities treated them that they did not like. They organized demonstrations against this treatment and knew enough about organizing that they were able to get large numbers of other drug users to take part in the demonstrations and were able to help other *Junkiebonden* to organize in other cities in the Netherlands and in nearby European countries.

Other groups were organized primarily as representatives of the clients of treatment centers. The BMG in Groningen is a small group that put out a magazine for members of other *Junkiebonden* and for professionals in the drug field. Still another, the MDHG in Amsterdam, struck me as being in a kind of halfway status. It had been organized by people whose primary interest was in drug policy reform, and the paid staff were nonusers, but a number of ex-users and current users were in its leadership and in its volunteer groups. (Interestingly, in the 1980s and 1990s, I would often hear or read other researchers who had visited Amsterdam refer to the MDHG as a "junkie union" and proceed on as if it were the leading example of such drug users' organizations. This certainly was not the opinion of most users' group activists at the time.)

I also met a member of one of the Australian users' groups near the end of 1986 when I went to Geneva for the first meeting to set up what became the World Health Organization Multicentre Study of Injection Drug Users and AIDS. I learned that the Australian government had arranged for and funded every state to have a drug users' organization to work against HIV and to provide policy advice to public health agencies, as well as a "national peak body," the Australian Intravenous League (AIVL) to perform these tasks at a national level and to help the state organizations. AIVL and the other Australian groups have been major players in the world of drug user organizing ever since they were set up. Jude Byrne, for example, the head of AIVL, served as the chairperson of the board of the International Network of People Who Use Drugs for many years. Long before that network was set up, however, the Australians went to international AIDS and harm-reduction conferences to help in efforts to coordinate the activities of drug users' groups around the world. They also took part in various programs to help users' groups get established in Asia and Pacific Islands countries. (I have written several papers with activists in the Australian groups, such as Jude Byrne and Annie Madden, and with other user activists as well, such as Eric Schneider, but in some cases cannot divulge that they are such in a public journal).[6,7]

Within a year, I had obtained funding to set up an HIV prevention program in New York that involved helping drug users to organize.[4,7-14] The results of the New York study, and of my qualitative analyses of various visits I made to drug users' groups in Australia and the Netherlands, helped drug users around the world to organize and to become an important part of street-level HIV, hepatitis C virus, and overdose prevention efforts and to be important advisors on national public health and drug policy issues in a number of countries.

In the United States, the level of repression and stigmatization of drug users has been extremely high during the entire period of the HIV epidemic. This has meant that organizing users' groups here has been very difficult. When the North American Syringe Exchange Network had its conferences during the late 1980s and onward for about 20 years, or during the conferences of the Harm Reduction Coalition once they began, there would often be a meeting to discuss organizing that was going on. I would usually be invited to these meetings. In general, we were very careful not to publicize who had attended, because some of the attendees were not publicly known as drug users. For example, some of them were leaders of syringe exchanges whose existence might be threatened if it were known that their leaders were drug users. In contrast with Canada, where the Vancouver Area Network of Drug Users had a public office and had meetings of scores of members that I attended at various times, and where there were other users' groups in most major cities, there were only sporadic periods in a US city when there were users' groups that publicly proclaimed themselves to be such. (It was public, however, that there were US or North American networks of drug user activists who held various meetings.)

At one point during the mid- to late-1990s (I think), I began to work on plans for a grant proposal to the US National Institute on Drug Abuse for research on drug users' organizations in comparison with outreach projects. I developed the beginning of this proposal and then discussed it with a number of NIDA program officials. They made it clear that they and NIDA were not interested in funding such a project. Other efforts to get funding for such research have also come to naught. One such effort was led by Jurgen Anker, who had conducted some research on this topic for the Nordic countries and organized meetings to try to do a project on a Europe-wide (or even wider) basis. This never came to fruition, unfortunately.

During the ensuing years, I took part in a number of meetings of users' groups and of people trying to set up users' groups in different locations in the United States, Canada, Australia, Europe, and elsewhere. I did this as a trusted nonuser, because I have never in my life taken any illegal drug or, indeed, smoked tobacco—although I was exposed to an enormous amount of tobacco smoke, and some other forms of smoke, in the course of these activities—without, I might add, ever feeling high as a result. Interacting with these users' groups and their members has been one of the most rewarding parts of my many decades in the field. I made many friends among these groups who remain dear friends today.

At this stage, there are user groups on every populated continent. They are coordinated by the International Network of People Who Use Drugs and by the International Network of Women Who Use Drugs. Regional groups also exist. This includes some large groups in East Africa and smaller ones in other parts of Africa; many groups in Asia and the Pacific; some in the Middle East and North Africa region; many in Europe, including Eastern Europe; and some in Latin America. A number of groups in both the US and Canada are open about being users' groups.

Their interests include HIV and hepatitis C prevention and care, but also include overdose prevention, drug treatment policy, police policy, drug policy reform, and the legalization of drug use, among others. The groups at the international level have listserves and other forms of electronic communication and host frequent and healthy debate on issues such as the role/oppression of women drug users and of drug users who are members of indigenous peoples, the best terminology to use in discussing issues about drug use and people who use drugs, and various aspects of how people who use drugs can both enjoy drugs and remain socially, legally, and physically safe while doing so.

Finally, let me reflect on how my involvement with and knowledge of drug users' groups has shaped my thinking. First, during most of the more than 30 years I have been in this field, it has helped me to understand that drug users are people with ideas and experiences that are critical for researchers and policymakers to understand. They are not just patients or clients who attend "drug abuse treatment programs" where they dutifully express their ideas in "treatment speak" so that they can get access to methadone or other resources. Nor are they people dependent on public health agencies or even harm-reduction organizations to think for them or to represent them. They are individuals with a wide variety of thoughts about drug use, art, politics, and anything else you want to name. Some of them are wiser than almost anyone in the drug research field; others are equally foolish.

In terms of the substantive issues around HIV/AIDS, working with drug users has taught me that when professionals set up outreach or other programs to teach drug users about HIV/AIDS, the people who use drugs often know far more about the field than do those who aim to teach them. This is not always true. When new scientific discoveries are made, someone has to make the new knowledge available to drug users. One of my current projects has spent considerable effort on this in terms of what is known about viral loads and transmission rates in the first year after a person becomes infected. In doing this, we rely on drug users to be able to learn the materials and then to teach other people who use drugs about them.[15,16]

Relatedly, we have studied concepts of "intravention," in which people who use drugs provide safety and health messages and knowledge to other people in their communities. We later realized that intravention can be thought of as the active process by which social norms are promulgated and maintained.

Finally, my work with drug users' organizations has helped me remember that HIV and related issues, as well as drug policies, are part of a wider society. In my experience, from my high school days on, from the early Civil Rights movement through to today, activism and social movements have been the driving force behind most positive changes in social policy. This has been true with HIV as well, as embodied in the activism of gay men, of the heroes who first established syringe exchanges in the United States and elsewhere when this was illegal or stigmatized, and of the activists who have forced the extension of antiretroviral treatment throughout the world. My work with users' groups has helped me find ways to bring this understanding into almost all of my work in the field. It has sustained me when my spirits have flagged, and when I have met defeats (such as when it became clear that no institute in the National Institutes of Health would fund research of heterosexual and mixed-group sex events and their role in HIV transmission and prevention no matter what priority score I got). It has helped me remember that top-down organizations and policies and programs, no matter how well intentioned and no matter who organizes or leads them (including myself), can become forms of oppression and that we need to work constantly against this happening.

I have worked with many extremely capable researchers, many of them probably far smarter than I have ever been. Nonetheless, I feel that much of what I have contributed to the field has sometimes gone beyond what some of these smarter researchers could see. This is because I built my understanding on the dialectical concept that the oppressed and exploited think and fight back, and that the goal of a researcher is often to build on what they know and help move it forward using the tools of research that might be less available to activist organizations.

Acknowledgments

This paper is attributable to support from the Community AIDS Prevention Outreach Demonstration, National AIDS Demonstration Research grant DA05283, and National Institute on Drug Abuse grant P30 DA11041 (Center for Drug Use and Research) and grant DP1 DA034989 (Preventing HIV Transmission by Recently Infected Drug Users).

References

1. Friedman SR, Des Jarlais DC, Sotheran JL. AIDS health education for intravenous drug users. Health Educ Q. 1986;13(4):383–93.

2. Friedman SR, Jarlais DC, Sotheran JL, Garber J, Cohen H, Smith D. AIDS and self-organization among intravenous drug users. Int J Addict. 1987;22(3): 201–9.

3. Friedman SR, de Jong WM, Des Jarlais DC. Problems and dynamics of organizing intravenous drug users for AIDS prevention. Health Educ Res. 1988;3(1):49–57.

4. Friedman SR, de Jong W, Rossi D, Touze G, Rockwell R, Des Jarlais DC, et al. Harm reduction theory: users' culture, micro-social indigenous harm reduction, and the self-organization and outside-organizing of users' groups. Int J Drug Policy. 2007;18(2):107–17.

5. Friedman SR, Casriel C. Drug users' organizations and AIDS policy. AIDS and Public Policy. 1988;3(2):30–6.

6. Friedman SR, Southwell M, Bueno R, Paone D, Byrne J, Crofts N. Harm reduction—a historical view from the left. Int J Drug Policy. 2001;12(1):3–14.

7. Friedman SR, Schneider E, Latkin C. What we do not know about organizations of people who use drugs. Subst Use Misuse. 2012;47(5):568–72.

8. Dziuban A, Friedman SR. A gap in science's and the media images of people who use drugs and sex workers: research on organizations of the oppressed. Subst Use Misuse. 2015;50(4):508–11.

9. Friedman SR. Theoretical bases for understanding drug users' organizations. Int J Drug Policy. 1996;7:212–9.

10. Friedman SR. The political economy of drug-user scapegoating—and the philosophy and politics of resistance. Drugs: Educ Prev Pol. 1998;5(1):15–32.

11. Friedman SR, Sufian M, Curtis R, Neaigus A, Des Jarlais DC. AIDS-related organizing of intravenous drug users from the outside. In: Schneider E, Huber J, editors. Culture and social relations in the AIDS crisis. Newbury Park, CA: Sage; 1991. p. 115–130.

12. Friedman SR, Des Jarlais DC, Neaigus A, Jose B, Sufian M, Stepherson B, et al. Organizing drug injectors against AIDS: preliminary data on behaviorial outcomes. Psychol Addict Behav. 1992;6(2):100–6.

13. Jose B, Friedman SR, Neaigus A, Curtis R, Sufian M, Stepherson B, et al. Collective organization of injecting drug users and the struggle against AIDS. In: Rhodes T, Hartnoll R, editors. AIDS, drugs and prevention: perspectives on individual and community action. London: Routledge; 1996. p. 216–233.

14. Latkin C, Friedman S. Drug use research: drug users as subjects or agents of change. Subst Use Misuse. 2012;47(5):598–9.

15. Friedman SR, Downing MJ, Jr., Smyrnov P, Nikolopoulos G, Schneider JA, Livak B, et al. Socially-integrated transdisciplinary HIV prevention. AIDS Behav. 2014;18(10):1821–34.

16. Vasylyeva TI, Friedman SR, Smyrnov P, Bondarenko K. A new approach to prevent HIV transmission: Project Protect intervention for recently infected individuals. *AIDS Care.* 2015;27(2):223–8.

Social and Behavioral Science

We're From the Government
and We're Here to Help You

BARRY S. BROWN

A S THE TRAGEDY OF AIDS and its impact on the drug-using population became increasingly evident through the mid-1980s, the National Institute on Drug Abuse (NIDA) deliberated on the role it should assume in response to the crisis. While there was strong feeling on the part of some members of NIDA's executive staff—such as Marvin Snyder, the Institute's director of research—that NIDA could and should make HIV a focus, the prevailing view was that the disease, however concerning, was essentially another of the public health risks to which drug users were vulnerable. As such, it was seen as appropriate for NIDA to lend what support it could to treatment programs coping with the epidemic, but the Institute evidenced no interest in developing a services research program to develop and test strategies for HIV/AIDS prevention. Consequently, NIDA sponsored a meeting for state directors of substance abuse treatment programming, inviting directors from states most vulnerable to the disease, to permit discussion of issues and a sharing of strategies. Additionally, NIDA staff compiled collections of articles from the professional literature describing findings and program initiatives relative to HIV/AIDS, which were to be mailed to state directors of drug abuse treatment programs and selected others with substance abuse treatment responsibility.

At best, these activities constituted a limited response to an expanding crisis. In a later instance in which NIDA elected to take a more expansive role, it ran into unexpected and significant opposition from the Reagan administration. With issues in transmission of the disease still incompletely understood, NIDA developed a brochure describing what was known about transmission and what individuals could do to protect themselves. In accordance with Administration concerns about certain language, care was taken to use terminology intended to make it more palatable to the administration, such as "the exchange of body fluids" rather than a less oblique discussion of sex. The then-acting director of NIDA, Jerry Jaffe, who had earlier been chosen by President Richard M. Nixon to be the nation's first drug czar, and I met with the individual sent from the Reagan White House to confer with us about the brochure. I was the chief of the Community Research Branch at NIDA. Conferring, as it turned out, consisted of our being directed to bury the brochure. No reason was given and we were simply informed that the administration did not want it issued. A short time later, a seething Jaffe and I left this briefest of briefings.

Advent of HIV/AIDS Programming

In 1987, Congress appropriated funds specific to HIV/AIDS programming, and $90 million became available to NIDA to conduct AIDS-related research. An additional $10 million was provided to other agencies, such as the Indian Health Service, allowing them to better serve the populations for which they had responsibility. NIDA directed $30 million to research modification and/or additions to treatment programming designed to respond to the HIV/AIDS epidemic, and $50 million was designated for the study of community-based outreach initiatives designed to contain the spread of disease to (and from) out-of-treatment injection drug users and their partners. The latter research program, under the imaginative and tireless leadership of George Beschner and with the strong support of Robert Battjes, led to a consortium of 41 related studies embracing 50 cities selected on the basis of risk for disease, as determined by rates of injection drug use and after approval of peer-reviewed applications.

The NADR Program

The resulting National AIDS Demonstration Research (NADR) program involved outreach programming such that workers, typically ex-addict paraprofessionals, recruited injection drug users in their home communities for the purpose of involving them in either of two intervention strategies. One strategy could be broadly characterized as behavior skills training/counseling and the other strategy as network-based behavior change. In the first strategy, outreach workers referred injection drug users to experienced counselors with training and expertise in HIV prevention techniques. In the second strategy, outreach workers inserted themselves into existing injection drug user networks and attempted to influence the thinking, attitudes, and behavior of the group and its members. All drug users were offered HIV testing and pre-test and post-test counseling. Additionally, all interventions relied on the capability of formerly addicted outreach workers to, at minimum, engage drug users who had rejected drug abuse treatment as a behavior change option. One can marvel at their success. More than 30,000 injection drug users and their sex partners were engaged over the life of the NADR program.

This was not the first time formerly addicted paraprofessionals were called on to respond to a crisis in drug abuse programming. Fifteen years earlier, when community-based treatment programming was introduced in hundreds of communities nationwide, paraprofessional and typically ex-addict staff were recruited, trained, and came to provide such effective services that national treatment evaluation studies were able to establish demonstrated reduction in drug use and criminal behavior of clients. And, in both the earlier and later instances, paraprofessional staff were largely shunted to the side when the crisis they had met was past.

The NADR program was not the first initiative to combat AIDS in the addict community. Important efforts were already under way in New York City and San Francisco; however, the NADR program, by virtue of its size and scope, quickly became the most significant initiative intended to contain the spread of AIDS through and from the injection drug user community. As such, it became subject to attack as an undesirable effort at "harm reduction" from some in the field concerned with what was seen as an implicit acceptance of drug use, given the instruction program staff provided in the safe use of injection drugs. More ominously, some on Capitol Hill were hostile to the program based, in significant part, on their conceptions of the moral good. In 1988, those legislators achieved passage of a law banning needle exchange as a strategy in HIV prevention, and there was concern on the part of those in the field that the distribution of bleach and/or other aspects of prevention programming were viewed with near equal distaste. The politics surrounding the national AIDS prevention program was to lead to my own curious exchanges with the press.

The Contentiousness of Needle Exchange

By the end of 1988, George Beschner was ready to call an end to a long and distinguished career, during which the development of a national HIV/AIDS prevention initiative had been just one highlight. I was asked to administer the program thereafter. A short time later, it came to light that one person employed under a NADR grant was spending a portion of his work time counseling at a needle exchange program. This appeared to be an illegal expenditure of federal dollars, and I judged that such activity could jeopardize the national outreach program, given the critics already in place on Capitol Hill. I sent a letter to the administrators of all NADR programs advising them that it was illegal to use federal funds to support needle exchange programs and warning them that any such activity threatened to undermine the whole NADR program. After my letter was shared with a member of the press, I received a call at home from a *New York Times* reporter wanting to explore my opposition to needle exchange.

I spent the better part of an hour trying to explain how my letter was intended only to protect a somewhat fragile program, that I had no personal animus toward needle exchange, and that it was essential we not appear to be breaking the law if we were to continue the AIDS prevention program. (Years later, I am happy to note that Richard Needle and I steered NIDA's first needle exchange grant through NIDA's Advisory Council.) To the reporter's everlasting credit, she elected to forgo the story and protect the program.

I wasn't as fortunate with a second *New York Times* reporter a good deal later. In this instance, the reporter wanted to do a feature story on the NADR program. I corrected her on one misunderstanding about the program, emphasizing it was not a needle exchange program, then reaffirming that point several times during our conversation. Nonetheless, the story that appeared in the *Times* described NIDA's groundbreaking needle exchange program. The story appeared on Christmas weekend, and while some might regard it as the equivalent of coal in my stocking, it was in truth a godsend that, if it was to appear at all, it arrived coincident with an extended weekend. I was able to contact the reporter's editor, explain the situation, and have a retraction printed in the *Times* before the deputy director of the Alcohol, Drug Abuse and Mental Health Administration (ADAMHA) could call me, as he did, to ask, "What the hell did you do now, Brown?"—or words to that effect.

Unsung Heroes

Beschner not only left behind a brilliantly innovative program, he also made available to me a dedicated and creative staff, including Gloria Weissman, who made unparalleled contributions in work with women at risk, Alberto Mata, Ro Nemeth-Coslett, and Rebecca Ashery. Later, we were joined by Richard Needle, Jeanette Johnson, Gary Palsgrove, Susan Coyle, and Helen

Cesari, all of whom further strengthened the team's capability. We also found powerful allies at the Centers for Disease Control (CDC), in particular Steve Jones and Steve Bowen, who, unsolicited, provided continuing support and encouragement to the NADR program and, when the capacity for distributing bleach was being challenged, supplied the influence that insured its continuing availability.

Establishing Credibility for Intervention Models

We determined that if the outreach program were to influence programming beyond the life of the demonstration grant period, it would be essential to establish its credibility with as rigorous a study as was feasible. As part of that that effort, we needed manuals describing the implementation of strategies being tested. To that end, all grant-funded programs were required to develop detailed implementation manuals for the particular interventions they had developed. All programs were also subject to evaluation protocols making use of identical baseline and follow-up instruments. To make certain the outreach program findings would be widely known and the credibility of the AIDS prevention program well established, investigators were encouraged to publish their findings individually.

Additionally, NIDA gathered articles for a volume of studies examining issues in the behavior change process and describing NADR outcomes obtained in terms of the reduced needle and sex risk behaviors.[1] To further establish the credibility of our research findings, NIDA published a paper summarizing the NADR program's positive outcomes, thereby putting its imprimatur on a report of the overall effectiveness of the AIDS outreach prevention program.[2]

Two intervention models were found particularly effective. One model involved a behavioral counseling approach developed by Fen Rhodes and colleagues[3] in Long Beach, California. The other model involved a network-based approach centered in addicts' own communities developed by Wayne Wiebel and colleagues[4] in Chicago. Further, a core NIDA model making use of counseling in association with outreach and HIV testing was found to dramatically reduce needle and sex risk, leading to the development of an implementation manual for that intervention by Susan Coyle.[5] With these manuals, and the availability of investigators and their service provider colleagues, NIDA would again work with the directors of state drug abuse treatment agencies—this time to have them select community-based provider organizations in their state that might best benefit from training in any of the three interventions and to select the intervention(s) most appropriate to programs in their state. In all, 17 training workshops were conducted, involving over 300 programs and more than 500 participants.

Life After Demonstration for NADR

The HIV/AIDS prevention projects known as NADR were funded as a demonstration research program and were intended to run the five-year course prescribed for that type of program. At a meeting in the office of the director of ADAMHA, it was announced that the assistant secretary for health had reaffirmed the five-year limit to the program. When opinions were solicited from the group, only one person expressed dissatisfaction with that decision.

The following day, I was to provide testimony to the National Commission on AIDS, the congressionally mandated body charged with recommending AIDS policy. I was told I would be providing the research findings from the NADR program. Given my sophistication about political process, I believed that was, in fact, the sole interest of the commission members. I got my first clue that there was an additional agenda when, about halfway through my report, I was politely asked how much more I had to present. When I had finished, I was questioned by the commission at length and repeatedly about whether the AIDS prevention outreach program was to be continued. My report, that effort was being made to convince directors of state drug abuse programming to continue funding outreach efforts in their states, did not generate enthusiasm, and the commission made clear its dissatisfaction with the program's termination. The message was received. Within a week, ADAMHA found the funds to support another iteration of the NADR program.

A short time after informal discussion between NIDA and California Congressman Henry Waxman's staff, language was inserted in legislation authorizing block grant funding to the states for mental health and substance abuse treatment, stipulating that programs were to provide AIDS prevention outreach where injection drug users could not access treatment. The regulations for that legislation, as prepared by the Center for Substance Abuse Treatment, specified the three models for use as those for which NIDA had earlier provided training.[6] The center used the same three models for its own outreach program after the agency was awarded $10 million in seed money for AIDS prevention.

Let Us Not Forget the Ground Troops

While I have emphasized NIDA's role because that is the perspective available to me and the activity with which I am most familiar, the NADR program's success was, of course, the work of many hands. In addition to the dedicated and talented people at NIDA with whom it was my privilege to work, the investigators and program managers for the NADR programs recognized the significance of their mission and acted accordingly. They were charged with combating a disease with well-established lethality and to act on behalf of a body of clients who excited little public concern or sympathy, and they conducted themselves with appropriate compassion and skill. And it was, of course, the outreach and clinical staffs who were called upon to be in direct and frequent contact with those clients and who were engaged daily in life-saving practice. Their success was reflected in the numbers compiled by programs and reported by NIDA. The numbers are unquestionably impressive, but numbers alone fail to capture the partner protected from AIDS, the child born free of disease, or the individual enabled to live free of disease and empowered to reclaim his or her life. Outreach workers and clinical staffs, alone, could see the effects of their efforts on individuals whose lives were protected and on communities made safer. They are the heroes of the struggle to halt the spread of disease within communities many would choose to ignore. It was left to the rest of us to support and quantify their success.

References

1. Brown BS, Beschner GM, editors. Handbook on risk of AIDS. Injection drug users and sexual partners. Westport, CT: Greenwood Press; 1993.

2. National Institute on Drug Abuse (NIDA). The National AIDS Demonstration Research (NADR) Project: effectiveness of AIDS outreach intervention/prevention research project on out-of-treatment injecting drug users. Rockville, MD: NIDA; 1994.

3. Rhodes F. The behavioral counseling model for injection drug users: intervention manual. Rockville, MD: National Institute on Drug Abuse; 1993.

4. Wiebel WW. The indigenous leader outreach model: intervention manual. Rockville, MD: National Institute on Drug Abuse; 1993.

5. Coyle SL. The NIDA HIV counseling and education intervention model: intervention manual. Rockville, MD: National Institute on Drug Abuse; 1993.

6. US Department of Health and Human Services. Substance abuse prevention and treatment block grants. Fed Regist. 1993:17064.

First AIDS Grant, First Interviews With AIDS Patients, First Syringe Exchange Politics, First Syringe Research

DON C. DES JARLAIS

PROLOGUE: THIS IS A "first" story of how I began my research on AIDS among persons who use drugs. It is also a story of the courage and altruism of persons dying from or at risk for AIDS.

AIDS among persons who inject drugs (PWID) was first reported in December 1981 by Masur et al.[1] six months after the report of the first cases of AIDS among men who have sex with men was published in the *Morbidity and Mortality Weekly Report* from the Centers for Disease Control in June 1981.[2] At that time there was almost no interest in AIDS at NIDA (the National Institute on Drug Abuse). There were only a handful of cases of AIDS among PWID and the institute was focused on drug use itself, with little or no attention paid to adverse consequences of drug use other than the continuing use of drugs.

Dr. Charles Sharp, a NIDA project officer, was, however, passionately concerned about AIDS. Dr. Sharp oversaw NIDA research on amyl nitrates ("poppers"), which were used to enhance sex by many men who had sex with men. While it seemed very unlikely that use of poppers (or any other drug) would lead to the severe immunosuppression seen among people with AIDS, Charlie Sharp strongly believed that AIDS was of great scientific importance and that it should be the subject of NIDA-funded research. Charlie visited New York City in the summer of 1982, convened a group of researchers and clinicians, and made a persuasive case that a research study of AIDS among persons who inject drugs was urgently needed.

I attended that meeting with Charlie Sharp. At that time, I was the deputy director of the Bureau of Research of the New York State Office of Drug Abuse Services. I was responsible for the day-to-day supervision of the epidemiology and program evaluation research conducted by the bureau and was personally working on studies of methadone maintenance treatment (with Vince Dole and Marie Nyswander)[3] and the Addicts Who Survived oral history project (with David Courtwright and Herman Joseph).[4]

The group agreed with Charlie Sharp that we should write a grant proposal to study AIDS among PWID. I had been following the scientific literature on AIDS and was intrigued by the newness of the phenomenon. While people who use drugs had always had high rates of various illnesses, there clearly had never been anything like AIDS. The severe immunosuppression and wasting syndrome were quite distinctive. I volunteered to write the proposal and serve as the principal investigator for the grant.

Writing the proposal was quite challenging. At the time there was very little known about AIDS and extremely little known about AIDS among people who injected drugs. The only thing known with certainty was that AIDS was uniformly fatal—no one was known to have recovered after a diagnosis of AIDS. It seemed likely that a previously unknown infectious agent was the cause of the syndrome, and that this agent was probably transmitted through sharing injection equipment and male-with-male sex. The first priority of the research would be to confirm—to the greatest extent possible—that the causative agent was transmitted through sharing injection equipment. However, not everyone who had shared injection equipment had AIDS, so that it was likely that there were specific injection behaviors that were associated with a greater chance of developing AIDS. Knowledge of such specific behaviors might provide strategies for reducing the likelihood that persons who injected drugs would be able to avoid developing AIDS. It was also plausible that there could be other factors, possibly including use of specific drugs, that might be important in the development of the severe immunosuppression seen in the diagnosed cases of AIDS. The proposal thus had to be state of the art in drug use epidemiology, drug use behavior, infectious diseases, and immunology. Fortunately, our research group did contain expertise in all of these areas (Drs. Mike Marmor, Robert Maslansky, Donna Mildvan, Tom Spira, and Stan Yancovitz). The New York City Health Department, under Commissioner Dr. David Sencer, and with Drs. Pauline Thomas, Rand Stoneburner, and Mary Cumberland, also contributed important flow cytometry laboratory resources, AIDS surveillance data, and critical expertise. The research design was a case-control study—to compare PWID with AIDS to PWID without AIDS on a great variety of demographic, behavioral, and immunologic factors. Dr. Sam Friedman joined the research team in 1985 and has made numerous invaluable contributions to the research.

The grant ("Risk Factors for AIDS," DA R01 003574), submitted in late 1982, was funded on the first submission, and the research started in late 1983. During that time, the number of identified cases of AIDS among PWID was doubling every six months. Beth Israel Medical Center, which had the largest substance use treatment program in the country and a large AIDS treatment program, was the primary site for conducting the study. Dr. Robert Newman, the president of Beth Israel, was a strong supporter of both substance use treatment and AIDS treatment.

While developing the proposal, with the questionnaire items and immunological variables, was intellectually challenging, interviewing persons with AIDS was emotionally intense. The persons with AIDS were interviewed in hospitals in the city. Again, at this time, there was no certainty regarding how AIDS was transmitted. This uncertainty led to considerable shunning and mistreatment of persons with AIDS within medical facilities, drug treatment programs, and correctional facilities. Interviewing persons with AIDS in the hospital required taking appropriate precautions (masks, gloves, protective garb, being extremely careful in handling biological specimens) and making a firm decision that I would treat these patients with dignity and respect.

The most important reason for the emotional intensity of these initial interviews, however, was the response shown by the subjects. They were literally dying, and dying from an AIDS opportunistic infection was a very bad way to die. The AIDS patients I was interviewing were typically emaciated, had difficulties breathing, and were in great pain. The interview I was administering was quite long—about two hours—as we wanted to explore the various ways in which people may have contracted the disease and what roles their drug use may have played in the development of the syndrome. There were many detailed questions that required considerable mental effort to answer. Answering the detailed questions was also emotionally difficult for these AIDS patients. They had to reflect upon their many years of drug use, knowing that they were soon going to die from their drug use.

Despite these worst possible conditions for conducting an interview, the research participants put great effort into answering the questions as completely and accurately as possible. I could see them fight losing consciousness, fight the pain, and exhaustively search their memories to answer the questions. They clearly knew they personally had nothing to gain by participating in the interview. But they were making supreme efforts in the hopes that the research might lead to preventing AIDS in others.

It has now been over thirty years since those initial interviews with AIDS patients. During that time, I have had many confirmations of the courage and altruism of persons who use or have used drugs to reduce HIV transmission in the community. This has included sharing information about HIV and AIDS, developing new social norms against sharing injecting equipment, working in syringe exchange programs (including times when this risked arrest because the programs were not legally approved), conducting secondary exchange out of syringe exchange programs, and leading advocacy efforts to improve health and social services. The actions of persons who use drugs have been critical in the movement toward adopting a public health/evidence-based/harm-reduction perspective on psychoactive drug use.

At a personal level, the courage and altruism shown by the AIDS patients in those first interviews created an enduring sense of obligation for me to do my utmost to reduce HIV transmission and other harms associated with psychoactive drug use. In both my research and in my policy work, I have felt that my ultimate responsibility was to persons who used drugs and to their communities.

These initial interviews were completely consistent with the hypothesis that the new disease was transmitted through the sharing of needles and syringes. The AIDS patients reported extensive sharing of needles and syringes. The supply of needles and syringes was severely limited in New York City at the time. Prescriptions were required to purchase needles and syringes, and possession of "narcotics paraphernalia" was a crime in itself. The supply was sufficiently limited that sharing was considered an altruistic act, helping out one's peers. Many injections occurred in "shooting galleries," places where one could rent a needle and syringe for injecting. These needles and syringes would then be rinsed—to prevent clogging, not to remove pathogens; the rinse water was used repeatedly. The needle and syringe would then be used by the next person who came to the shooting gallery.

In addition to conducting interviews and CD4 T cell testing with AIDS patients and monitoring AIDS diagnoses among people who injected drugs, we were working with the Centers for Disease Control on developing an antibody test. The CDC was working with Drs. Luc Montagnier and Françoise Barré-Sinoussie of the Institut Pasteur to develop an antibody test for the lymphadenopathy-associated virus that they had recently discovered. We sent samples from our research subjects to Dr. Tom Spira at CDC, who arranged to have them tested with the new antibody test that the CDC was developing in collaboration with Montagnier and Barré-Sinoussie.

The results of our first antibody testing of PWID in New York were quite disturbing. As expected, the antibody testing confirmed the association of

LAV with AIDS. However, more than half of the PWID without AIDS were antibody positive.[5] We also collaborated with Dr. Mary Jeanne Kreek of Rockefeller University to establish the history of the epidemic among PWID in New York City. Mary Jeanne and Dr. David Novick had conducted research on PWID with liver disease at Beth Israel Medical Center in the mid-to-late 1970s. They had stored samples that we then tested for anti-HIV. These showed rapid transmission of the virus among PWID, with prevalence rising from under 10 percent in 1978 to over 50 percent by 1981.[6] An additional very disturbing finding came from our collaboration with Dr. Rand Stoneburner of the New York City Department of Health. We examined deaths among PWID in the city and found a very large number of deaths from unusual infections, such as extrapulmonary tuberculosis, that coincided with the AIDS epidemic but were not included in the official case definition of AIDS. The case definition was developed primarily through studies of men who have sex with men and thus did not include the full spectrum of infections that were occurring among PWID. If these excess deaths were considered as AIDS cases, then the number of AIDS deaths among PWID would be twice as high.[7]

Thus, our early findings revealed a very disturbing picture—the AIDS virus could spread very rapidly among PWID, could reach very high prevalence, and led to a much larger spectrum of fatal illnesses than was previously known.

First Stories of Risk Reduction Among PWID, Self-Initiated Behavior Change Among PWID, and Syringe Exchange

Our studies and other studies finding substantial HIV prevalence among PWID in other cities showed substantial prevalence, e.g., over 30 percent in Amsterdam[8] and 60 percent in Scotland,[9] and created a great urgency to reduce HIV transmission among PWID. Much of my career has been spent studying risk and harm reduction among people who use drugs, but I want to recount just two first stories here.

As part of my responsibilities in the Research Bureau of the New York State Office of Drug Abuse Services, I oversaw the field research unit. This unit worked in the community and monitored trends in street drug use in the city. PWID in New York learned about AIDS quite early. There was extensive media coverage of AIDS in the early to mid-1980s, there were visible cases of people with AIDS in the community, and AIDS was much discussed among PWID. PWID made the analogy to hepatitis B and concluded that the disease was transmitted through sharing needles and syringes. This led to increased demand for clean syringes, as PWID were trying to reduce their chances of getting AIDS.[10,11] PWID in New York were changing their behavior prior to any official public health efforts to reduce HIV transmission in the group.

Starting syringe exchange programs, in which used—potentially HIV contaminated—needles and syringes could be exchanged for clean needles and syringes was an early obvious idea for reducing HIV transmission among PWID. A syringe exchange had actually been established in Amsterdam prior to HIV testing in the city. The exchange was implemented after a major pharmacy in the city center stopped selling syringes to drug users. The exchange was thus originally implemented to reduce transmission of hepatitis B among PWID but was greatly expanded after the HIV testing was conducted.

I visited Amsterdam in the fall of 1985 to begin a research collaboration with Roel Coutinho of the Amsterdam health department and to visit the Amsterdam exchange. I was impressed with the exchange, which was operated by the *Junkiebonden* (drug user unions; see the chapter by Friedman in this book). I returned to New York with hopes of establishing a syringe exchange program in New York City. I worked with the City Department of Health to plan a pilot study of syringe exchange in the city. Dr. Sencer wrote a memorandum to Mayor Koch in support of a pilot program. The memorandum was leaked to the police department, who effectively vetoed the program. Koch concluded that "syringe exchange is an idea whose time has not come and will not come."

Epilogue

While this first attempt at syringe exchange research could not overcome political resistance, I was soon conducting syringe exchange research with Holly Hagan and Dave Purchase in Tacoma, Washington, and Kathy Oliver in Portland, Oregon, and internationally through the World Health Organization Multi-site Study of HIV and Injecting Drug Use.[12] New York eventually implemented a large-scale syringe exchange program in 1992, and I evaluated the effectiveness of those programs.[13,14] I have continued policy work on harm reduction as a member of the US National Commission on AIDS, the New York State and New York City commissions on AIDS, the Ending the Epidemic Task Force in New York State, and various national and international advisory groups.

My first grant has been renewed continuously and is now in years 31 to 35, studying "Getting Close To Zero" new HIV infections among people who use drugs in New York City. Getting close to zero new HIV infections has taken much too long, but it is the fitting outcome for those first research participants whose courage and dedication to helping their peers has been the most vivid memory throughout my career.

References

1. Masur H, Michelis MA, Greene JB, Onorato I, Vande Stouwe RA, Holzman RS, et al. An outbreak of community-acquired *Pneumocystis carinii* pneumonia: initial manifestation of cellular immune dysfunction. N Engl J Med. 1981;305:1431–8.

2. CDC. *Pneumocystis* pneumonia—Los Angeles. MMWR 1981;30:250–2. https://www.cdc.gov/mmwr/preview/mmwrhtml/june_5.htm

3. Dole VP, Nyswander ME, Des Jarlais DC, Joseph H. Performance-based rating of methadone maintenance programs [letter]. N Engl J Med. 1982;306(3):169–72.

4. Courtwright D, Joseph H, Des Jarlais DC. Addicts who survived: an oral history of narcotic use in America, 1923–965. Knoxville: University of Tennessee Press; 1989.

5. Spira T, Des Jarlais D, Marmor M, Yancovitz S, Friedman S, J G, et al. Prevalence of antibody to lymphadenopathy-associated virus among drug-detoxification patients in New York. N Engl J Med. 1984;311(7):467–8.

6. Des Jarlais DC, Friedman SR, Novick DM, Sotheran JL, Thomas P, Yancovitz S, et al. HIV-1 infection among intravenous drug users in Manhattan, New York City, from 1977 through 1987. JAMA. 1989;261:1008–12.

7. Stoneburner R, Des Jarlais D, Benezra D, Singh T, Sotheran J, Friedman S, et al. A larger spectrum of severe HIV-1-related disease in intravenous drug users in New York City. Science. 1988;242:916–9.

8. R van den Hoek JA, Coutinho RA, van Haastrecht HJA, van Zadelhoff AW, Goudsmit J. Prevalence and risk factors of HIV infections among drug users and drug-using prostitutes in Amsterdam. AIDS. 1988;2(1):55–60.

9. Robertson R, Richardson A. Heroin injecting and the introduction of HIV/AIDS into a Scottish city. J R Soc Med. 2007;100:491–4.

10. Anderson W. The New York needle trial: the politics of public health in the age of AIDS. Am J Public Health. 1991;81(11):1506–17.

11. Normand J, Vlahov D, Moses LE, editors. Preventing HIV transmission: the role of sterile needles and bleach. Washington, DC: National Academies Press; 1995.

12. Des Jarlais D, Hagan H, Friedman S, Friedmann P, Goldberg D, Frischer M, et al. Maintaining low HIV seroprevalence in populations of injecting drug users. JAMA. 1995;274(15):1226–31.

13. Des Jarlais DC, Marmor M, Paone D, Titus S, Shi Q, Perlis T, et al. HIV incidence among injecting drug users in New York City syringe-exchange programmes. Lancet. 1996;348(9033):987–91.

14. Des Jarlais DC, Perlis T, Arasteh K, Torian LV, Beatrice S, Milliken J, et al. HIV incidence among injection drug users in New York City, 1990 to 2002: use of serologic test algorithm to assess expansion of HIV prevention services. Am J Public Health. 2005;95(8):1439–44.

The Development, Testing, and Implementation of an Information–Motivation–Behavioral Skills Model for the Prediction and Promotion of HIV/ AIDS Preventive Behavior

JEFFREY D. FISHER AND WILLIAM A. FISHER

O NE OF US (Jeff) was born on April 23, 1949, and by some miracle the other (Bill) was born on April 23, 1952. After years of intense sibling rivalry—occasioned in part by sharing the same bedroom and in larger part by our parents' desire for us to be best friends—we finally began to collaborate, first helping each other to decode if not fully understand the true, intensely interesting dynamics of our family of birth, and later in endeavors with more potential to benefit society.

After completing our undergraduate degrees, September 1974 found us overlapping for a year as social psychology doctoral students at Purdue University, studying under the late and beloved Professor Donn Byrne. Jeff had spent his first summer at Purdue funded by Donn's grant from President Lyndon Johnson's Commission on Obscenity and Pornography, directed by Donn to write pornography and assess whether married people were more aroused by it in written form, in a movie, or in their imaginations. When Bill arrived, Donn was studying the more prosaic issue of how to increase condom use to prevent pregnancy, and we collaborated with him on this and other projects. In retrospect, our first joint publication, "Consumer Reactions to Contraception Purchasing," published in 1977,[1] probably reflected our inclination to apply social psychological theory in the service of sexual health promotion.

In 1985, 10 years after graduating from Purdue, and some 32 years ago, at the tender age of 35, Jeff was lazing in a hammock in his yard in rural Connecticut reading the *New York Times*, when he encountered a worrisome article about AIDS. It reminded Jeff, a social psychologist, of his work on sexual risk behavior with Bill and Donn in graduate school. Jeff called Bill to discuss it. We talked intently about AIDS throughout summer 1985. AIDS was having a devastating effect on the gay and drug-using communities. It had become clear that this "plague" was not going away, and there was increasing hysteria that it would spread to the heterosexual community.

Some of our earlier joint research focused on how to interrupt the sexual behavior sequence and introduce condom use to decrease other sexually transmitted infections (STIs). And Bill had continued to do significant work on human sexual risk and preventive behavior after graduate school, while some of Jeff's work in the mid-1980s had been on people's potential to change behavior across a broad array of contexts. We began to ruminate on how we might apply a distinctive social psychological approach to combat AIDS. A curse (or a distinct benefit) of growing up in the 1960s was a pervasive need to believe one's work could have potential to help change the world and significant motivation to attempt to do so.

Thanksgiving Dinner, 1985

Our first "in person" meeting on our new research focus was after Thanksgiving dinner in our parents' dining room (Figure 25.1), where we brought our social psychological roots and shared social consciousness to the AIDS problem. We initially adopted twin research foci, involving understanding and promoting the voluntary adoption of AIDS preventive behavior (APB) and constructively managing the widespread fear of AIDS that fueled occasionally horrific discrimination against people living with HIV (PLWH). We had received a few small grants to study AIDS fear, AIDS knowledge, and AIDS prevention under the supposition that these constructs might be related.

At the time, the state of AIDS prevention science consisted largely of best guesses by non-psychologists who thought the best way to prevent it was simply informing the public about AIDS (e.g., "Abstinence or condom use can prevent becoming infected") or scaring the bejesus out of them ("You could die from AIDS if you're not careful"). We conducted our initial research on fear of AIDS, AIDS knowledge, and APB in Connecticut and Ontario, Canada. We soon learned that there was more to AIDS prevention than simply informing and scaring people.

We explored extant social psychological theories that could be used to conceptualize AIDS prevention but felt all were missing a critical piece or two of the puzzle. We read the few published efficacious AIDS prevention interventions for clues, collected more data, began to make presentations and write papers, and submitted larger grant proposals on our hypotheses and findings. In 1987, we gave our first joint presentation of our AIDS research. In 1988 Jeff published his first major paper on AIDS[2] in *American*

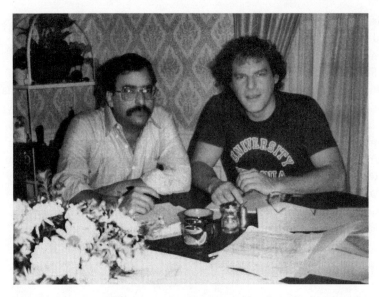

FIGURE 25.1. William A. Fisher (*left*) and Jeffrey D. Fisher after Thanksgiving dinner, 1985, Columbus, Ohio. Photo by Helen Fisher, their mother.

Psychologist on the effects of reference-group social influence on APB. That year, Bill coauthored a paper on AIDS risk behavior in *Journal of the American Medical Association*. Also in 1988, we received our first significant external funding from the Social Sciences and Humanities Research Council of Canada for a project titled "Fear of AIDS and APB." In 1989 we received our first large grant from the US National Institute of Mental Health (NIMH) for a project titled "A General Technology for AIDS Risk Behavior Change." A major collaborative research enterprise was initiated.

Breakfast, and a Model Is Born

A pivotal event occurred at the 1988 Vermont Conference on the Primary Prevention of Psychopathology, devoted that year to psychological approaches to preventing AIDS. Why it happened over breakfast we couldn't tell you, but a couple of ideas crystallized about the suspected missing puzzle pieces. First, we realized that most social psychological theories applied to APB were more or less solely motivational in nature. While several were exceptionally well articulated and empirically supported (for example, the Theory of Reasoned Action[3]), purely motivational approaches did not address the need for easy-to-enact, script-like prevention information that

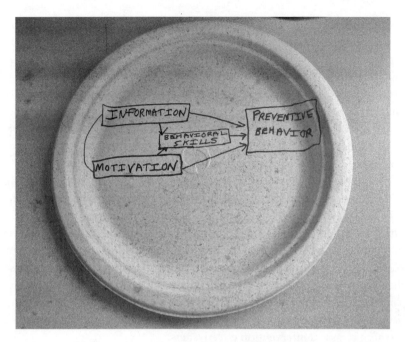

FIGURE 25.2. The legendary paper plate depicted above is a reconstruction; the original has been lost somewhere in our files or possibly recycled. The Information–Motivation–Behavioral Skills (IMB) model of AIDS-preventive behavior first appeared in print in *Psychological Bulletin* in 1992.[7] Photograph by Jeffrey D. Fisher. Used with permission.

could be readily deployed by an individual, nor did they provide even basic information about transmission and prevention needed in early stages of epidemics.[4] Other work[5,6] alerted us to the critical role of the individual's behavioral skills in performing complicated and often novel APBs, from anticipating sex and the need for prevention to discretely acquiring condoms, negotiating their use, employing them correctly, and having a sense of self-efficacy in doing so. The pieces fell into place. We scribbled the results on a paper plate, which comprised the humble beginnings of our Information–Motivation–Behavioral Skills (IMB) model of AIDS risk and prevention (Figure 25.2).[7]

IMB Model of AIDS Preventive Behavior

At the simplest level, the IMB model asserts that essential determinants of initiation and maintenance of APB are easy-to-enact, script-like AIDS prevention *information*, personal and social *motivation* to act on what one knows about AIDS prevention, and objective and perceived *behavioral skills* for enacting APBs effectively.[8,9] Because APB often involves initiation and maintenance of complicated, novel, and socially challenging behavioral skills, the IMB model holds that, in general, AIDS prevention information and AIDS prevention motivation work through the application of AIDS prevention behavioral skills to result in the enactment of APB (Figure 25.2). More than two decades of empirical research supportive of the IMB model are described in detail, most recently by Fisher, Fisher, and Shuper.[9]

In addition to using the IMB model in multiple prediction studies to understand the determinants of APB, we were urgently committed to applying it in APB promotion interventions and articulated a three-step approach.[8] First, we would perform elicitation research[8,10] to clarify the information, motivation, and behavioral skills assets and deficits in a target population. Next, we would implement empirically targeted interventions to addresses the information, motivation, and behavioral skills needs identified in elicitation research, with respect to the most pressing AIDS risk behaviors identified in the target population. Finally, we would conduct rigorous evaluation research to assess intervention effectiveness.

Time Passed and Things Happened

Critical to our progress was NIMH support for our Information-Motivation-Behavior model–based AIDS prevention prediction and intervention research for 25 years. Studies have confirmed IMB model predictions that information, motivation, and behavioral skills are critical determinants and account for substantial variance in the production of APB, and that the effects of information and motivation generally work through, and are mediated by, an individual's level of behavioral skills. Moreover, under specified conditions, information and motivation may have direct effects on preventive behavior.[9] We've also supported the IMB model assumption that the specific content of its information, motivation, and behavioral skills constructs and their relative strength in predicting APB vary as a function of the particular APB and population in focus. These variations, captured in elicitation and model testing research and reviewed in Fisher et al.,[9] are critical to tailoring optimally effective interventions. In terms of interventions, we and others have designed, implemented, and evaluated a very substantial number of successful IMB model–based AIDS prevention interventions worldwide, targeting almost every group at risk for contracting or transmitting HIV. For an extensive review, see Fisher et al.[9] We are pleased that some of these have been widely disseminated.

In addition to APB, specific IMB models have been articulated for conceptualizing and increasing/promoting the following: health behavior, broadly defined; medication adherence, including in clinical drug trials and adherence to a postsurgical regimen; healthcare-seeking and maintenance in care; health-related Internet use; obesity prevention; diabetes self-management; and cancer screening, among others. In many of these contexts, the assumptions of the more specifically articulated IMB models have been confirmed through correlational model testing and experimentally based intervention research.[9]

Experiencing Success With Help From Our Collaborators

What is most important about our work on the IMB model of HIV prevention—our major joint focus for 32 years—is that with colleagues we were able to articulate, test, and confirm the predictions of a new model for understanding and preventing HIV transmission that has been successfully utilized worldwide in interventions to increase APB and in the process save lives. Most all of our work on APB has been described in detail elsewhere.[9] Thus, we devote the remainder of this chapter to detailing some important experiences we had along the way and some of the lessons learned about life and science that we have not, until now, had a forum to recount.

What We Learned

First, Kurt Lewin[11] was absolutely right—there is nothing as practical as a good theory. We have experienced firsthand that good social psychological theories can be remarkably useful in gaining insight into the dynamics of, and in intervening to solve or change, even the most intractable human problems and behaviors. Good theories can absolutely be the basis of powerful behavioral interventions that can save human lives, as demonstrated by many HIV prevention researchers over the years. Sadly, well-validated theories have been too infrequently used to improve public health or for any other sort of "real world" benefit, something we hope will change dramatically.

Second, people (including ourselves, our research participants, and our staff) can regularly do things they thought were impossible. For example, during graduate school, Donn Byrne quickly taught his graduate students we could do things that we formerly believed were not possible. He gave us an intense, immersive mentorship and training experience and seemingly impossible responsibilities, and he (and we) regularly found we could function like junior faculty members. He didn't teach this to us by *telling* us we could do the impossible, but rather by *expecting* us do the seemingly impossible and to succeed at it. We, in turn, have engendered the belief that much of what might initially seem impossible is actually possible in generations of PhD and postdoctoral students, staff, and others.

For instance, the physicians in our HIV prevention-for-positives interventions initially thought significant HIV risk behavior change might be impossible for their patients. They also thought it might be impossible for them to interact as equals with patients in assisting them to change their AIDS risk behavior, a precondition for physicians' effective use of motivational interviewing[12] to help patients change behavior. Our physician collaborators almost always learned that their initial beliefs about the limitations on what they and their patients could accomplish individually and together were incorrect. The fact that given the right conditions, people can do things they and others thought were impossible is demonstrated daily in our research. Deeply believing that very substantial behavior change is possible and being able to identify the key active intervention ingredients to spawn it are key to success in the field of health behavior change.

Third, when you "get into the trenches" to change seemingly intractable human problems, you can come into contact with wonderful as well as difficult and even despicable people, places, and practices. Working over the years in the United States and Africa on HIV prevention, we met courageous giants of love and compassion in the medical, public health, and advocate professions and among HIV patients and the public (and too rarely, but occasionally, in the government and religious professions) who persisted in helping those infected and affected by HIV against all odds and doing the impossible daily. We experienced this early in the HIV epidemic, and it continues today. Surprising to us at first, for more than 25 years we generally have found officials at the NIMH (our funders) and the grant review process itself to be fair and equitable, even in a political context sometimes unsupportive to HIV research. Off the record, NIMH officials even gave us advice about how to change the wording of the abstracts of our funded grants so they wouldn't be defunded by Congress during the administration of George W. Bush and how to widely disseminate the intervention materials they had funded and we had validated, without becoming lightning rods for political attack.

While our colleagues, fellow scientists, and administrators who were not HIV prevention researchers were generally quite supportive of our work, on occasion a few of our colleagues displayed prejudice and ignorance. Some were upset, for example, when we filmed several people living with AIDS in the psychology building for a research video at a time in the epidemic when it was well known that HIV was not spread casually. Others questioned the university provost's plans to construct a facility for research on HIV prevention, which people living with or at risk for HIV might participate in, adjacent to a student dormitory complex. Once, when one of our babysitters took her three young children to a local mall food court, she found herself seated next to three university professors having a discussion about a colleague (one of us) who was apparently (a) a married, closeted homosexual with children who (b) likely had AIDS and who was (c) "cashing in" on HIV since it was a new and "easily funded" research area. To do this sort of work, one has to develop thick skin.

Sometimes one's detractors can even include those that one is trying to help. At one point in the epidemic, we realized that AIDS prevention research focused almost exclusively on uninfected individuals and scrupulously avoided research involving nonstigmatizing and supportive HIV risk-reduction interventions for PLWH, who are the only ones who can infect others. Reviewing all published HIV prevention interventions, we found[13] that only 59 of 898 focused on HIV prevention among PLWH. NIMH funded us to do some of the initial, supportive, HIV risk-behavior change research to lower HIV transmission risk behavior among PLWH. When one of us presented our research plans for "prevention with positives" research to support the wishes of most PLWH—that the epidemic should stop with them—at a meeting of the National Association of People with AIDS in San Francisco, he was told unequivocally that they did not "need, or want, AIDS policemen." However, strong voices from southern US women of color took the opposite tack—"If Fisher can prevent one woman from getting infected, he should do it"—which won the day. He was then taken out for drinks by the group at a local San Francisco drag bar and, as they say, a good time was had by all.

In South Africa, ignorance and/or objections to our prevention-for-positives research took other forms. About the time of the inception of our project, the president of South Africa unfortunately began to maintain publicly that poverty and malnutrition (not HIV) cause AIDS and that antiretrovirals were poison. This was antithetical to the success of our research, which aimed to increase condom use among PLWH to prevent HIV transmission and contain the epidemic. Moreover, when we began conducting this research in KwaZulu-Natal (KZN)—with permission from the KZN Department of Health (KZNDOH)—neither American nor South African researchers working in the area welcomed us. A powerful American HIV medical researcher and his colleague attempted to shut our project down by complaining to the KZNDOH that it would contaminate their (hoped-for) future research sites "should one of their postdocs want to run a study there someday," showing a primitive and counterproductive sense of research territorially, a distain for behavioral research, and no concern whatsoever about denying local residents a potentially life-saving intervention. And a group of South African researchers working in the same locality tried to scare us away by informing us (rather hysterically, and incorrectly) about how terribly dangerous it was to travel and to send research staff out in the area, when they were (apparently) really worried they might lose employees to our new project and preferred we work elsewhere to prevent this.

After we have rigorously demonstrated the efficacy of one of our HIV prevention interventions, we offer our standard-of-care control clinical sites free training in our intervention protocols so they can implement the intervention with their patients. More than once, we've had control sites decline to spend the time to learn to implement a proven intervention that could have saved lives. Over the years, we learned, sadly, that while most scientists and practitioners are wonderful people, some are unfortunately more interested in themselves than in broad-based scientific progress or in the overall well-being of the population they are apparently attempting to benefit.

In addition to occasional bad behavior by scientists and practitioners, in our work on AIDS in Africa we sometimes encountered levels of human degradation, poverty, and death that were initially impossible to fathom; a profound lack of resources; and occasionally downright stupidity. What we encountered the next day was sometimes worse, and these experiences changed us forever. We saw hospitals with AIDS wards located on the fifth floor, necessitating that terribly sick, very weak people walk up five flights of stairs. The elevator was invariably broken, and when it worked it was nicknamed the "TB express" since sick, coughing PLWH with tuberculosis (TB) or multiple-drug-resistant TB took it with healthy staff, family, and guests. When we arrived on the fifth floor, we could see hundreds of people dying under awful conditions. When we traversed it again after a brief meeting with a doctor or staff members, some patients had died.

In urban and rural clinics, we encountered crowded patient waiting rooms with hundreds of PLWH waiting long times for appointments, some coughing with TB, and without open windows or airflow, increasing the potential for TB transmission. We saw clinics filled with sick, often immune-compromised people for which the only source of water was a well situated immediately outside that had a metal cup attached to a string, which everyone shared. If there was anything good about some of these profoundly moving and distressing conditions, it is that some comprised fairly "low hanging fruit" that was relatively easy to change, with profoundly favorable health implications. In low-resource settings or elsewhere, one should always look first for the low-hanging fruit.

Fourth, when you get into the trenches with intractable human problems, you can be profoundly emotionally affected in many ways. We had other profoundly moving experiences that affected us emotionally and which are part of working with seemingly intractable human problems. One was filming a series of videos entitled *People Like Us*[14] in the psychology building during our first NIMH grant. We filmed six young, attractive high school—and college-aged PLWH who had never been particularly risky in their behaviors but had contracted HIV from their relationship partners, through the same risk behaviors practiced by many heterosexually active adolescents. The videos were informed by Festinger's[15] social comparison theory, which argues that the most psychologically meaningful (and motivating) comparisons are with similar others. In effect, confronting students with others just like them (or those they would like to have sex with), who did what they do but who contracted HIV, could powerfully motivate behavior change. The speakers represented the diversity of the high school and college populations and each told their stories, let us deeply into their lives, and described their illness, their suffering, and how others had treated them. One was banned from Thanksgiving and Christmas dinner with their family and had to eat alone after everyone else. Others had been deathly ill and almost died. All of us at the filming cried. We realized we were creating something bigger than us and our particular project and distributed the video widely. Within a year, each of those appearing in *People Like Us*[14] had died. For years, we got letters from teachers and others who had shown the video, asking what had become of them. Every time we showed the video on campus, we received calls from local HIV testing sites asking if we had shown the video again, as it was that effective in motivating behavior change.

Many of those we met with AIDS over the years are still with us emotionally. When we began to work in Africa, we saw graveyards crowded with makeshift shallow graves and sticks with names scrawled on them. Families had to sneak into the graveyards by dark to bury their dead because they couldn't afford a burial plot or a decent burial. In Africa, we visited profoundly ill PLWH in their simple homes, living in deep poverty but full of life and determination. When we returned from Africa after every trip, we felt guilty.

Fifth, doing research has sometimes become unnecessarily difficult and painful for the researchers. Doing this sort of work is profoundly difficult, and researchers do it because it is important, not because it is fun. Grant review committees are often populated by folks more eager to show how critical they can be than to promote a conceptually compelling set of ideas that might make a difference. We've learned over the years the importance of the older, grayer, sometimes charismatic voices on review committees asserting the importance of not losing the big picture. When they are funded, grants almost automatically experience funding cuts each year, accompanied by requirements for more participants, more complex designs, lengthier follow-ups—all laudable but unfunded aims. Enough said.

Sixth, "just enough ego." Returning to our story, we reflect on how two brothers managed to work together for three decades and emerge not only still talking to one another but stronger for the struggle. We think the answer is in the informal "just enough ego" model that we've followed: just enough ego to assertively articulate one's conceptualization or approach, to sculpt and refine it in the back and forth of spirited discussion and criticism with our team; just enough ego to modify one's ideas, shift course, or cede to a better idea, when one emerges; just enough ego to get the two of us through every step of the way in the challenging but beautiful process of inventing, articulating, and implementing new ideas and new methods.

Biomedical Tsunami

We've pointed out that early efforts to contain HIV were spearheaded by professionals trained in medical but not necessarily behavioral science. The same could be said about the recent "Biomedical Tsunami" in HIV/AIDS prevention, a move to deemphasize behavior change and replace it with biomedical fixes generally involving "treatment as prevention." It is clear that antiretroviral therapy (ARV) can render an infected individual uninfectious, vastly reduce mother-to-child transmission, and reduce the likelihood of a risky individual being infected and that circumcising an adult male can markedly reduce his and his partner's risk of acquiring HIV. What has not yet been sufficiently realized is that these biomedical interventions are fundamentally behavioral interventions. Undergoing HIV testing, adhering to ARV regimens, and undergoing adult circumcision are examples of the "complex and novel behaviors required for HIV prevention" that may be driven or deterred by—guess what?—an individual's relevant information, motivation for acting on this information, and behavioral skills for practicing prevention. And let's not forget—deemphasizing safer sexual behavior while practicing biomedical HIV prevention strategies opens the door to other STIs, which, like HIV, can come out of left field. For all these reasons, safer sex interventions and sensitivity to the behavioral complexities of biomedical fixes will be necessary to prevent the continuation of this epidemic or the start of the next one.

In Retrospect

When we met for tea after dinner in 1985 to discuss HIV prevention research, we had no idea our emerging collaboration would ultimately contribute in meaningful ways to both the science and practice of HIV prevention, generate 127 joint publications and presentations and almost $25 million in NIMH research funding, permanently change our career paths, and persist for most of the remainder of our careers. The opportunity to engage in the world of ideas, to study the dynamics of unhealthy behavior, and to develop and test models that describe it and interventions to change it is an amazing privilege. We found that it helps to be a bit crazy in this line of work, with the costs of the cavalcade of human misery to keep you company, the academic machine highly inclined to reward short-term sexy but long-term low-impact work, and grant review committees sometimes too eager to, as Marty Fishbein once put it, "Eat their young." We do this work and encourage our students to do it, first because it is absolutely necessary; and second, because the application of behavioral science in this area is an outstanding context for the development and testing of sophisticated theory. The outcome variables, such as infection or death, will keep one both engaged and humbled.

Acknowledgments

To have been able to do our work at a critical juncture in the AIDS crisis, and to have had it supported by the NIMH for quarter century, is a privilege. To have had such wonderful employees, PhD students, post-doctorates, and colleagues—far too numerous to name—on our NIMH- funded projects over the years has been a further privilege. Each of these folks deserves a measure of the credit for any success we have had.

References

1. Fisher WA, Fisher JD, Byrne D. Consumer reactions to contraceptive purchasing. Pers Soc Psychol Bull. 1977;3:293–7.

2. Fisher JD. Possible effects of reference group-based social influence on AIDS-risk behavior and AIDS prevention. Am Psychol. 1988;43(11):914–20.

3. Fishbein M, Ajzen I. Belief, attitude, intention and behavior: an introduction to theory and research. Reading, MA: Addsion-Wesley; 1975.

4. Fisher JD, Fisher WA. Theoretical approaches to individual-level change in HIV risk behavior. In: Peterson J, DiClemente R, editors. Handbook of HIV prevention. New York: Kluwer Academic/Plenum Press; 2000. p. 3–55.

5. Bandura A. Self-regulation of motivation and action through goal systems. In: Hamilton V, Bower GH, Frijda NH, editors. Cognitive perspectives on emotion and motivation. Dordrecht: Springer Netherlands; 1988. p. 37–61.

6. Kelly JA, St. Lawrence JS, Hood HV, Brasfield TL. Behavioral intervention to reduce AIDS risk activities. J Consult Clin Psychol. 1989;57:60–7.

7. Fisher JD, Fisher WA. Changing AIDS-risk behavior. Psychol Bull. 1992; 111(3):455–74.

8. Fisher WA, Fisher JD. Understanding and promoting AIDS preventive behavior: a conceptual model and educational tools. Can J HumSex. 1992; 1(3):99–106.

9. Fisher WA, Fisher JD, Shuper P. Social psychology and the fight against AIDS: an information-motivation-behavioral skills model for the prediction and promotion of health behavior change. In: Olson J, Zanna M, editors. Adv Exp Soc Psychol: Elsevier; 2014. p. 105–193.

10. Fisher JD, Fisher WA, Aberizk. Elicitation Research Methods. In: Blanton H, Webster GD, editors. Social Psychological Assessment Methods. New York: Routledge; in prep.

11. Lewin K. The Research Center for Group Dynamics at Massachusetts Institute of Technology. Sociometry. 1945;8(2):126–36.

12. Miller WR, Rollnick S. Motivational interviewing: preparing people to change addictive behavior. New York: Guilford Press; 1991.

13. Fisher WA, Fisher JD, Kohut T. AIDS exceptionalism? The social psychology of HIV prevention research. Soc Issues Policy Rev. 2009;3:45–77.

14. Fisher JD, Fisher WA, Marks D. People like us [videotape]. Available from AIDS Risk Reduction Project, Department of Psychology, University of Connecticut, Storrs; 1992.

15. Festinger L. A theory of social comparison processes. Human Relations. 1954;7:117.

Out of Suffering

New Directions in AIDS Behavioral Prevention Research From a Personal Perspective

WILLO PEQUEGNAT

I WAS FORTUNATE TO WORK at the National Institute of Mental Health (NIMH) for 26 years, beginning during the early response to the suffering of men and women experiencing a disease no one understood (see also the chapter by Rayford Kytle). One afternoon in 1989 shortly after receiving my PhD, while wandering the halls of NIMH looking for an interesting job, I ran into the husband of the woman who had hired me at the American Psychological Association before I went to graduate school. I told him my story and he brightened. He introduced me to a woman who had just received funding for a new program to address research issues to study a mysterious new disease, and she needed staff. He reassured me that she was usually there late. I had a brief meeting with her and we seemed to click. She put me on a professional services contract and pitched me tasks to determine where I could make a contribution.

Because I had never worked for the federal government, I was clueless about the procedures to implement any of the tasks successfully. Not deterred, she gave me a second professional services contract and I successfully conceptualized a new research initiative. We were fortunate to develop a creative relationship with a network of gifted behavioral prevention investigators who guided NIMH's global HIV prevention research program.

We realized we were stewards of important funds and needed to ensure that they were invested carefully. During those early years, the NIMH AIDS program was receiving 10 to 15 percent funding increases. Spending that much new money requires vision, creativity, and commitment to ensure that the grant money would have the greatest impact. We therefore promulgated program announcements that solicited innovative AIDS prevention research that provided rigorous scientific data demonstrating that programs were both effective and cost effective and did not duplicate other studies. The program addressed behavioral issues that arose during different phases of the AIDS epidemic. During all of those phases in HIV behavioral prevention research, we were fortunate to have persons living with HIV as investigators, collaborators, and friends, because they brought the reality of the epidemic into focus, which in turn helped guide the urgent nature of our work.

In 1983, even before the routes of HIV transmission were fully understood, the federal government had begun to mobilize a response to this new public health threat. Public health officials suspected that AIDS was a social disease associated with sexual behaviors. However, federal support for sexual behavioral research had been terminated in the early 1970s because it was controversial in the Nixon administration. Consequently, no good prevalence data existed on the HIV-related risk behaviors of Americans, and few, if any, models for prevention of high-risk HIV-related sexual behaviors were available.

To develop effective population-specific prevention programs, it is essential to understand what people know, think, and do, which is why the early studies concentrated on collecting data on knowledge, attitudes, and behavior (KAB). To identify KAB patterns, investigators conducted studies with people exhibiting symptoms of the illness and those without symptoms. Studies also identified antecedent behaviors (such as drinking alcohol or sharing needles) and settings (such as bars, bathhouses, and shooting galleries) that place people at risk for HIV and other sexually transmitted infections (STIs). This period was characterized by multiple KAB studies for different risk groups and the legitimization of AIDS as a relevant area of behavioral prevention research.

The next major HIV research era occurred from 1986 to 1991 and was characterized by the activism of ACT UP (the AIDS Coalition to Unleash Power) that adopted the slogan "Silence=Death." We were so grateful for their advocacy, as this period changed forever the way the National Institutes of Health conducts research. For example, community advisory boards became valued and mandatory; investigators and others living with HIV participated in finding solutions for their disease; research subjects took their pills to chemists to break the blind nature of the studies; and persons suffering from HIV/AIDS demanded progress in research. Even the director of the National Institute of Allergy and Infectious Diseases acknowledged that some AIDS activists understood the biological mechanisms of the virus better than some of his lab scientists.

Zidovudine (AZT), a nucleoside reverse transcriptase inhibitor, was the first drug to show promising signs of efficacy. The pressure from desperate individuals suffering from AIDS resulted in the blind being broken early, and in 1987 the Food and Drug Administration approved AZT. Despite these breakthroughs, widespread fear and stigmatization persisted toward those at high risk for HIV/AIDS (especially gay and bisexual men). Unfortunately, this lack of accurate information about HIV transmission fostered growing support for policies that would restrict the civil liberties of individuals known to be HIV positive.

This lack of reliable data on risky sexual behavior continued to make it difficult to design effective behavioral prevention research. Despite resistance to public support of sexual behavioral research, NIMH was able to fund the National AIDS Behavioral Survey. Using a random digit dialing strategy to "cold call" potential respondents, the National AIDS Behavioral Survey demonstrated that Americans were less hesitant about answering explicit questions about their sexual behaviors than had been believed; only 17 percent of those contacted refused to respond to the survey.

By this time an antibody test had been developed and seropositive individuals could be distinguished from those who were seronegative, so it was possible to conduct comparative studies to identify predictors of seroconversion. Because of the public health imperative and insistence by AIDS activists, behavioral prevention research moved toward conducting single-site, single-population studies that tested proof of concept for prevention programs with at-risk seronegative persons to reduce their sexual and drug-use behaviors, such as unprotected sex or needle sharing. These interventions were based on social cognitive theory and delivered at the individual level.

Despite the advancements in behavioral and medical research, by 1994 AIDS was the leading cause of death among Americans aged 25 to 44. Between 1992 and 1997, research began to pay off. Having demonstrated that single-site behavioral prevention interventions work, the next phase involved conducting large randomized controlled trials with multiple populations and sites, using both behavioral (e.g., unprotected anal intercourse) and biological (e.g., seroconversion) outcomes.

While important work was being conducted at the individual level during this period, researchers also recognized that HIV could affect the entire family and that multiple family members and generations could be at risk or infected. To reduce HIV incidence, investigators developed additional HIV prevention programs at other than the individual level, including at the couple, family, community, and societal (media and policy) levels. Investigators demonstrated that behavioral prevention must be titrated to the risk behaviors and life context of at-risk individuals. For example, some people may benefit from brief interventions, whereas others may require a more sustained intervention. To facilitate this research, from 1990 to 2010 NIMH supported yearly conferences entitled "The Role of Families in Preventing and Adapting to HIV" in a different location around the country to bring together local service providers and prevention researchers to craft research to meet the needs of specific at-risk communities.

In 1995, highly active antiretroviral therapy (HAART) was introduced, with the first protease inhibitor, saquinavir. The following year, the Food and Drug Administration approved the first non-nucleoside reverse transcriptase inhibitor, nevirapine, and a viral load test to measure levels of HIV. These developments were able to revive many patients who were near death (known as the "Lazarus effect") and led to a 70 percent reduction in AIDS-related deaths.

Research then moved in a new direction by studying the role of voluntary counseling and testing (VCT). Although VCT had been viewed previously as an intervention to reduce HIV infection, with the advent of treatment, there was a new impetus for early HIV screening of at-risk populations to identify and treat people early in the infection, when they are the most infectious.

When introduced in 1993, the female condom was hailed as the first (dual-protection) female-controlled method capable of preventing both unwanted pregnancy and HIV infection. This, in turn, opened up research into behavior change in women, as women were taught to avoid risky situations and triggers for their risk behaviors and to negotiate female condom use.

During this period, a payoff occurred from another new research direction, community-level prevention research. This work was based on the theory of diffusion of innovation, a model to explain how new technological and behavioral innovations are initiated and become adopted by early adopters in community populations. Innovations often begin with "trusted leaders," whose actions and opinions lead other people to change their behaviors. This, in turn, modifies existing normative behaviors in a community. This strategy worked to change the norms of participants in high-risk community environments.

Research is necessary and important, but it is not sufficient to end an epidemic that causes such widespread suffering. While NIH had not viewed effectiveness studies (studies conducted in clinics under real-world conditions to determine if they are still efficacious) as their mission, NIMH investigators began to explore implementation in the public health system. Beginning in 1998, NIMH and behavioral prevention investigators partnered with the Centers for Disease Control to identify evidence-based interventions that were ready to be scaled up in public health clinics. CDC began a rigorous program called Diffusion of Effective Behavioral Interventions—which was modeled on the Good Housekeeping seal of approval—and began encouraging public health clinics that they supported to implement these evidence-based interventions. Besides evidence, another issue in the adoption process is cost effectiveness. Before clinics make a decision to use a Diffusion of Effective Behavioral Intervention, they want to know that they have the resources to successfully implement it. Investigators developed sophisticated methods for adapting and implementing these studies.

Randomized controlled trials demonstrated that evidence-based behavioral prevention programs reduced high-risk behaviors. The next step was to demonstrate, based on biological data, that these interventions actually prevented HIV infection, in settings with high HIV prevalence. NIMH began to support research in international settings where investigators could design studies with both behavioral and biological interventions and outcomes. The program funded research in some of the countries hardest hit by HIV/AIDS, such as in sub-Saharan Africa and India. Investigators used site visits as opportunities to develop collaborative research teams composed of in-country and US investigators. This strategy ensured that the research would be culturally congruent, address the risk factors in the community, and build an in-country research infrastructure and sense of ownership of the programs.

Multiple adherence issues can complicate HIV medication regimens, particularly for long-term survivors. In 2008, investigators began exploring treatment as prevention. Post-exposure prophylaxis (PEP) is a strategy that requires an individual to take an HIV medication after inadvertent exposure to HIV. Pre-exposure prophylaxis (PrEP) also uses HIV medications (such as Truvada) that are taken before exposure to prevent transmission. This is a good strategy for serodiscordant couples, where the individual who is HIV negative is continually exposed to HIV. However, several behavioral issues were associated with these strategies. Initially, for example, PrEP was viewed as possibly providing individuals with license to engage in more risky behavior. However, studies have demonstrated that this is not the norm; more studies are needed to determine associated risk behavior.

I feel fortunate that I arrived at NIMH at an opportune historical moment, which allowed me to be part of a team to contribute to ensuring that some NIMH-supported behavioral HIV prevention research moved in new and productive directions. I also made wonderful friends, worked with talented colleagues, traveled to amazing countries, and learned about different cultures. Despite our successful collaborative behavioral and biological research directions, the HIV/AIDS epidemic is continuing to cause suffering in international settings and there is still much to do in the United States. The baton has been handed to a new generation of researchers to design and test new research directions and innovative prevention strategies to alleviate the suffering of another cohort of people living with and affected by AIDS.

From the Many, One
A Collaborative Approach

CLYDE B. MCCOY, DUANE C. MCBRIDE,
AND ANNE JEANENE BENGOA

I T WAS ON A SUNNY Friday afternoon at the University of Miami School
of Medicine Grand Rounds that we first heard about a couple of unusual
cases that puzzled the physicians who presented them to the group in attendance. The first case involved a young Caucasian man of Northern European descent who had just been diagnosed with Kaposi's sarcoma, a cancer
that causes lesions to grow in the skin, in the lining of the mouth, nose, and
throat, and in the lymph nodes and other organs. The reporting physician
noted how unusual this was given that this disease was not known to exist
in this young man's age group or among those of Northern European decent. The second case involved a young man who had been diagnosed with
Pneumocystis carinii pneumonia (PCP), an illness that the attending physician said typically occurred among the very old and generally those living in
nursing home settings.

These cases puzzled the Grand Rounds group, who asked numerous
questions, including where the patients lived, where they had been, what
acute or chronic diseases they had, and who they interacted with. The
presenting physicians reported that there was nothing in the patients'
background that indicated any major acute or chronic diseases that would
suggest they would be susceptible to these illnesses that affected the elderly
and those with a compromised immune system. Almost an afterthought, it
was noted that neither of these young men appeared to have girlfriends that
visited them in the hospital.

At the advent of the search for the explanation of "this strange and per-
nicious disease," the University of Miami research centers, departments, and
schools attracted and organized a very effective multidisciplinary and interdisciplinary group. This allowed for a synergistic approach to determining

what the origins, consequences, and interventions should be for this new medical phenomenon that in the beginning went by multiple names, including Gay-Related Immune Deficiency (GRID) and Gay Disease.

A few medical centers around the country had begun to observe cases of individuals with this unusual disease spectrum. Some of the earliest signs included, for example, Kaposi's sarcoma or PCP or both. We were fortunate that in addition to our two research centers, the Comprehensive Drug Research Center (CDRC) and the Health Services Research Center (HSRC), we also worked with and had the support of our cancer center and many of the departments at the medical school, the school of arts and sciences, the School of Nursing, and the School of Business.

The research did not end at the University of Miami but has continued throughout the careers of many faculty and staff of both the CDRC and HSRC. The work of many staff members, and now department chairs, was a major driving force in the acquisition of various core grants, as was their participation in National Institutes of Health (NIH) grant review committees. Through these initial studies and support from numerous funding agencies and important stakeholders, crucial information regarding the HIV/AIDS epidemic became readily available, paving the foundation for future research.

The main objective of our group's multidisciplinary and interdisciplinary structure was to develop a collaborative partnership with all of the major stakeholders in order to obtain a comprehensive understanding of the emerging HIV/AIDS epidemic. The partnership paved the way for the creation of methods and practices to gather vital information regarding the new epidemic sweeping through south Florida. All of these efforts would not have been possible without the establishment of the National Institute on Drug Abuse (NIDA) in 1974, which set a precedent and priority for research on drug abuse and other health-related outcomes. More specifically, NIDA's support created the foundation for studying injection drug users, sex partners, and the spread of HIV/AIDS in Miami and its surrounding counties.

The clinical observations as well as the outreach efforts of mainly our drug/behavioral science and health services centers began piecing together the puzzle for the HIV/AIDS epidemic in Miami. This core group collaborated to provide the highest quality research, including studying the epidemiology of HIV/AIDS among drug users, developing and testing the efficacy of interventions to reduce high-risk behaviors, conducting field studies of drug paraphernalia, assessing the efficacy of bleach in eliminating the HIV virus from needles, and documenting the use and access to healthcare by

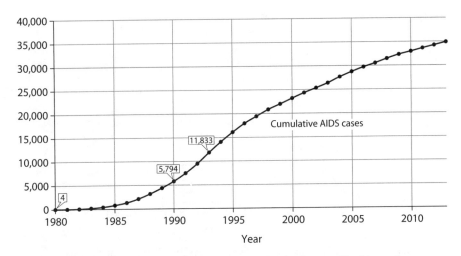

FIGURE 27.1. Cumulative AIDS cases, Miami-Dade County, Florida, 1980–2013. Graph produced with data from Florida Department of Health, Bureau of Vital Statistics.

drug users. Understanding the major risk factors, such as injection drug use and male-to-male sexual contact, through various disciplines highlighted the impact of such factors on the spread of HIV/AIDS.

Because each of us had access to and observations of different subpopulations and risk groups for various other diseases and behavioral/mental illness in addiction, this puzzle began taking shape in the mid-1980s. In fact, we were able to go back to 1981 and identify at least four cases that we would consider HIV/AIDS at these points.[1] By the late 1980s, some 2,500 cases were identified in Miami-Dade County, which doubled to 5,000 cases in 1990 and 10,000 in 1993 (Figure 27.1).[2]

Further, the number of HIV/AIDS cases identified and treated from 1994 to 2011 shows the impact of multidisciplinary and interdisciplinary efforts in the surveillance of the epidemic cases. From 1992 to 1994, a spike occurred in the number of HIV/AIDS cases and deaths, as shown in Figure 27.2, but negative health outcomes due to the HIV/AIDS epidemic have since continued to decrease due to these collaborative efforts. Surveillance efforts have allowed for consistent early detection of the HIV infection, which has created more efficient and effective treatment options that have further reduced the incidence of AIDS.

Eventually, we were able to link these sometimes seemingly independent observations and unlikely associations to various risk groups and spectra

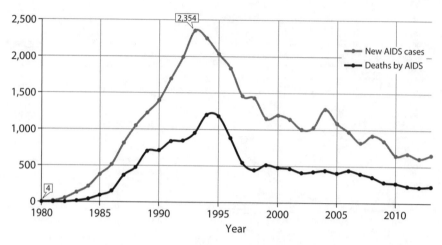

FIGURE 27.2. New AIDS cases and deaths by AIDS, Miami-Dade County, Florida, 1980–2013. Graph produced with data from Florida Department of Health, Bureau of Vital Statistics.

and to directly link the viral origins and disease outcomes of HIV/AIDS. We recognized that these various risk groups were involved in transmission vectors that seemed to direct to one risk group of gay individuals, particularly male-to-male transmission. The significant amount of ongoing research was facilitated by the various disciplines working together and recognizing that we were studying some of the same phenomena. Of course, virology and immunology, which had not yet seen their heyday, were of critical importance in recognizing this disease as being virally transmitted among risk groups and via common transmission vectors.

It was only through the multidisciplinary expertise of the collaborating team members from both the bench research and behavioral sciences that much of the crucial HIV/AIDS information was obtained. A multidisciplinary and interdisciplinary approach helped create a thorough and comprehensive understanding of the emerging epidemic. Through this comprehensive research network, a vast array of knowledge and accomplishments occurred, including discovering that HIV antibodies were in syringes and paraphernalia at shooting galleries,[3] documenting a wide series of HIV risk behaviors that facilitated moving toward risk-reduction approaches,[4,5-7] developing a protocol for needle cleaning and testing its efficacy,[8,9] working with NIDA and the Centers for Disease Control to develop and evaluate HIV risk-prevention protocols,[10] translating NIDA risk-reduction protocols to international settings,[8,12-16] and extending the

CLYDE B. MCCOY, DUANE C. MCBRIDE, AND ANNE JEANENE BENGOA

research of effective interventions to other classes of drug users, especially crack cocaine users.[17]

Given the richness of the database, multiple methods were used to capture the diverse populations impacted by the AIDS epidemic in this region. In addition to various statistical analyses, rich visualizations of the data have been utilized, such as maps, timelines, graphs, charts, and scattergrams. Independent analyses were made of the various subpopulations and a number of time series were generated to look at the wide variation of subpopulations by demographic and exposure groups affected over different periods.

Some observations in the number of new cases in Miami-Dade:

- AIDS cases went from only four in 1981 to nearly 35,000 in 2013.
- A gradual initial increase catapulted during the latter 1980s and early 1990s, reaching the highest annual number of new cases at over 2,300 cases in 1993 and 1994.
- A male-to-female ratio of approximately 3–4:1 has persisted since the mid-1990s as increases and decreases in both sexes shadow one another, with the exception of the Haitian population, where cases among females slightly outnumber cases among males.
- The number of female cases is approximately 20 percent of all people diagnosed with HIV (Figure 27.3).

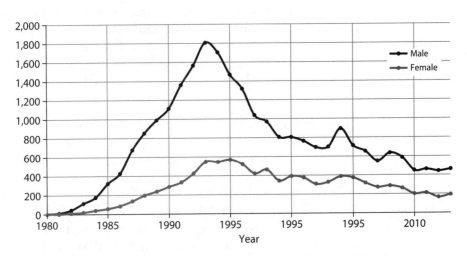

FIGURE 27.3. New AIDS cases by gender, Miami-Dade County, Florida, 1980–2013. Graph produced with data from Florida Department of Health, Bureau of Vital Statistics.

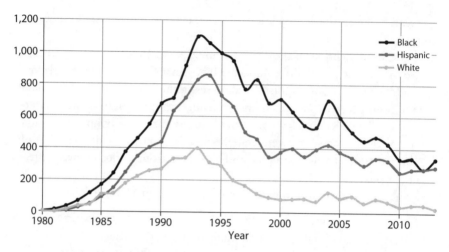

FIGURE 27.4. New AIDS cases by race and by year of diagnosis, Miami-Dade County, Florida, 1980–2013. Graph produced with data from Florida Department of Health, Bureau of Vital Statistics.

- The impact on minority populations has been much more severe at all time periods—Blacks/African Americans account for 50 percent and Latino/Hispanic populations account for about one-third of total cases (Figure 27.4).
- Among the Latino/Hispanic population, most cases were people from the Caribbean, specifically Cuba, Puerto Rico, and Haiti.
- Approximately 60 percent of all cases have ended in death.
- Increases in drug abuse risk, especially injection drug use, are noted throughout each time period, especially among injection drug users, who account for more than 40 percent of cases.[6]

Because of the interdisciplinary nature of the research spanning various departments, schools, centers, and universities, a collaborative network of university researchers, community agencies, drug treatment programs, hospitals, other healthcare entities (such as emergency departments), and other access points (such as correctional facilities and the medical examiner's office) were enabled to respond to the HIV/AIDS epidemic. Although the focus of this network was local, it soon became a statewide, regional, and national network. Also, the multiple faculty involved with HIV/AIDS research in these various departments and centers expanded their network to other universities, continued their HIV-related research, and contributed significantly to HIV epidemiology and prevention research in their new commu-

CLYDE B. MCCOY, DUANE C. MCBRIDE, AND ANNE JEANENE BENGOA

nities, as well as served on NIH AIDS-related grant review committees. In this sense, the initial efforts of the University of Miami influenced regional, national, and international HIV prevention efforts.

While challenges and obstacles have occurred, the rewards have far outweighed the difficulties in researching the HIV/AIDS epidemic from its emergence until the present day. Our experiences in the communities of Miami allowed us to develop new programs that corresponded closely with our efforts in addressing HIV/AIDS. Additionally, our research collaboration became actively involved with HIV/AIDS studies not only locally, but also nationally and internationally.

Acknowledgments

Shikha Puri and Alejandro J. Mendez.

References

1. Shultz JM, Elliott L, McCoy CB, Simmons JR, Lieb S, LaLota M, et al. Acquired immunodeficiency syndrome—Dade County, Florida, 1981–1990. MMWR Morb Mortal Wkly Rep. 1991;40(29):489–93.

2. Shultz JM, Damoulaki-Sfakianaki E, Metellus G, Gnesda D, McCoy CB. Acquired immunodeficiency syndrome in Miami/Dade County, Florida: the first 10,000 cases. Miami Medicine. 1995;66:17–22.

3. Chitwood DD, McCoy CB, Inciardi JA, McBride DC, Comerford M, Trapido E, et al. HIV seropositivity of needles from shooting galleries in south Florida. Am J Public Health. 1990;80(2):150–2.

4. McCoy CB, Inciardi J. Sex, drugs, and the continuing spread of AIDS. Los Angeles: Roxbury; 1995.

5. McBride DC, Freier MC, Hopkins GL, Babikian T, Richardson L, Helm H, et al. Quality of parent-child relationship and adolescent HIV risk behaviour in St. Maarten. AIDS Care. 2005;17 Suppl 1:S45–54.

6. McCoy CB, Metsch LR, Inciardi JA, Anwyl RS, Wingerd J, Bletzer K. Sex, drugs, and the spread of HIV/AIDS in Belle Glade, Florida. Med Anthropol Q. 1996;10(1):83–93.

7. McCoy CB, McCoy HV, Senk C, Bengoa AJ, Mendez AJ. Analyzing the AIDS epidemic from 1981–2013 in metropolitan Miami: National Institute on Drug Abuse International Forum; 2015.

8. McBride DC, Inciardi JA, Surratt HL, Terry YM, Van Buren H. The impact of an HIV risk-reduction program among street drug users in Rio de Janeiro, Brazil. Am Behav Sci. 1998;41(8):1171–1184.

9. McCoy CB, Shapshak P, Metsch LR, Rivers JE, McCoy HV, Weatherby NL, et al. HIV-1 prevention: interdisciplinary studies on the efficacy of bleach

and development of prevention protocols. Arch Immunol Ther Exp (Warsz). 1995;43(1):1–9.

10. McCoy CB, De Gruttola V, Metsch L, Comerford M. A comparison of the efficacy of two interventions to reduce HIV risk behaviors among drug users. AIDS Behav. 2011;15(8):1707–14.

11. McCoy CB. Institutionalization of drug abuse research in academia—one professor's view. J Drug Issues. 2009;39(1):reflections.

12. McCoy CB, McBride DC. HIV Research within the Global Context. Urban Health. 2005;82:2–4.

13. McCoy CB, Metsch LR, Page JB, McBride DC, Comerford ST. Injection drug users' practices and attitudes toward intervention and potential for reducing the transmission of HIV. Med Anthropol. 1997;18(1):35–60.

14. McCoy CB, Lai SH, Metsch LR, Wang XR, Li C, Yang M, et al. No pain no gain, establishing the Kunming, China, Drug Rehabilitation Center. J Drug Issues. 1997;27(1):73–85.

15. McCoy CB, McCoy HV, Lai S, Yu Z, Wang X, Meng J. Reawakening the dragon: changing patterns of opiate abuse in Asia, with particular emphasis on China's Yunnan Province. Subst Use Misuse. 2001;36(1&2):49–69.

16. McCoy CB, Rodriguez F. Global overview of injecting drug use and HIV infection. Lancet. 2005;365(9464):1008–9.

17. McCoy CB, Weatherby NL, Metsch LR, McCoy HV, Rivers JE, Correa R. Effectiveness of HIV interventions among crack users. Drugs and Society. 1996;9(1–2):137–54.

Historical Perspectives

The Beginning of Science in the HIV Epidemic

Eureka Moments

ROBERT C. GALLO

U SUALLY WE DATE THE BEGINNING of scientific exploration into an area with information derived from laboratory experiments. With AIDS, that is not the case, as the science emerged first from keen observation. To my thinking, the first key scientific observation came from clinicians who recognized the decline in CD4 T cells, which in turn gave some of us the notion that the cause of AIDS involved the direct impact on the development of, or lifespan of, the CD4-positive T lymphocyte. The second critical observation came from epidemiology and the championing of conceptual epidemiological clues formulated by James Curran, who became the director of the AIDS program at the Centers for Disease Control (CDC). Curran made us aware that there were well-defined risk groups, such as groups within a certain concentration (for example, the island of Haiti) and groups that had strong interpersonal connections and sexual contacts (particularly at that time and almost solely known at that time among the gay community), and eventually also defined high risk for people receiving blood transfusions or other blood products, especially hemophiliacs who received plasma combined from large numbers of donors, as well as intravenous drug addicts. Soon thereafter, Curran and other epidemiologists identified babies born to mothers who had AIDS as being at risk of contracting AIDS.

Yet, at the time, innumerable ideas for what caused AIDS were posited, and frequently they had little do with infectious disease. For example, one of the leading early theories was that AIDS was caused by amyl nitrate (or "poppers"), used as a sexual stimulant. This was proposed by investigators at the Food and Drug Administration but subsequently was modified by them as a limited needed factor for Kaposi's sarcoma. This idea had little credibility as to a sole cause of AIDS because the risk groups noted above were not always associated with the use of this drug. Another popular non-infectious theory was autoimmunity, which was based on rough sex transmitting leukocytes from one individual to another and the recipient reacting against these leukocytes with an immune response that eventually attacked the recipients' own cells, which, in turn, for some unknown reason led to depletion of the CD4 T cells. This idea gained traction among some leading immunologists in the United States, and it may even have been presented as a leading theory at a 1983 meeting at Cold Spring Harbor Laboratory. Ultimately, this theory suffered the same drawbacks as the amyl nitrate idea, as one could argue that rough sex has been around for a few million years and AIDS was new. However, from the start, Curran was proposing the notion of a new infection and probably a virus. I know this because it was his lectures in late 1981 and early 1982 at the National Institutes of Health (NIH) that steered me into AIDS research.

The years just before (the late 1970s) had been the most tranquil and rewarding that I had experienced. By the late 1970s, we had discovered the first human retrovirus, a long-time controversial subject that many derided as not plausible because of multiple prior failures and because of some scientific arguments that humans could not be infected by retroviruses. The one we discovered, which we called Human T cell Leukemia Virus-1 (HTLV-1), causes leukemia, usually in young adults, as well as a fatal spastic neurological disease and sometimes a variety of more modest disorders likely based on autoimmune phenomenon, including modest *immune deficiency*. As the start of the 1980s we also discovered a second human retrovirus, HTLV-2, which is very similar to HTLV-1 but for reasons not completely clear not so pathogenic.

When Curran first talked at NIH, he described a small number of patients, and though I thought it was interesting, it certainly wouldn't move me away from our leukemia research anytime soon. Yet, in early spring 1982, he gave a second lecture and it became very clear that this disease was reaching serious epidemic proportions. Curran queried, "Where are the virologists?" demonstrating that he was already thinking of a new virus. I felt he was looking at me when he asked that question, and when I returned to my laboratory across the NIH campus I thought maybe we could contribute something, because we had considerable expertise in culturing (growing cells in laboratory settings) human blood–derived T cells.

In 1976, we had discovered one of the first cytokines, now known as interleukin-2 (IL-2) but originally called T cell growth factor (TCGF). The consequence of that discovery gave us strong expertise in growing human T cells, especially CD4-positive T cells, and growing cells is of immense help in finding any new virus. Because it was CD4 T cells that were in decline and presumably might be the cells targeted by any new agent, we presumably had an edge. After multiple discussions, Max Essex—my friend and collaborator of many years at the Harvard School of Public Health—and I hypothesized that AIDS might be caused by another human retrovirus. We believed this because HTLV-1 and HTLV-2 happen to target CD4 T cells and HTLV-1 could cause minor immune suppression. We also knew that these viruses were transmitted by blood, sex, and from mother to infant in milk. Consequently, a variant of those viruses, perhaps also arising in Africa—as the evidence suggested HTLV-1 and HTLV-2 did, from an ancient transmission from chimpanzee to humans—was most likely the cause. Chimpanzees have viruses very similar to HTLV-1/HTLV-2 known as simian T-cell leukemia viruses. The basic idea was that AIDS may be caused by another retrovirus, different from HTLV-1 and HTVL-2, but presumably in the HTLV family—a putative HTLV-3. Among the many theories, this was the only one that bore fruit, but it was not completely accurate because HIV is not a "brother" of the HTLVs but rather a "cousin." As we soon learned, it belongs to a different category of retroviruses. This was quite astonishing in view of the fact that it took so long and was so difficult to prove that humans had one retrovirus; to then find a different subfamily of human retroviruses was remarkable.

In May 1982, my colleagues and I carried out our first experiments designed to follow this hypothesis. The group in France, led by Luc Montagnier, reported a retrovirus that seemed to be different from HTLV-1 and HTLV-2. I helped them by providing antibodies to distinguish what they had from HTLV-1 and HTLV-2 and by the method protocols for growing T cells with IL-2. I reviewed their paper, which showed a retrovirus isolate that also convinced me was neither HTLV-1 nor HTLV-2. It came from a patient with lymphadenopathy, a disease of the lymph nodes in which they are abnormal in size, number, or consistency. This was one patient and the virus could not be grown in substantial amounts, so it could not be easily characterized or used for an applicable blood test in any significant manner. Consequently, the group in France did not claim it was the cause of anything other than possible lymph node enlargement (as Montagnier later proposed in a Cold Spring Harbor paper), nor could they, as there was no linkage to AIDS.

Finding a virus particle and demonstrating that this exact virus with its characteristics defined is the cause of a disease, particularly one as complex as AIDS, is neither straightforward nor simple, nor does it involve a similar pattern of thinking or technology as finding a virus. Demonstrating the cause of AIDS to the scientific community would be particularly difficult because, as everyone now knows, AIDS develops only after multiple years and physicians and health workers were not accustomed to asking what someone did a couple of years ago or what their interesting exposures were multiple years ago. Moreover, by the time a person had AIDS they had many other infections. Which one was the cause?

Another difficulty, which is not often recalled, was quite acute. AIDS patients were not so plentiful and often were not even allowed in some institutions. Even samples of AIDS tissues were often forbidden. And most troubling of all, by the time a person had AIDS they had hardly any T cells in their peripheral blood. If the virus was lurking in some of those T cells, it was going to be extremely challenging to find it.

In their first sample, the French group fortunately received a lymph node biopsy rather than blood. The idea came from clinicians Willy Rozenbaum and Jacques Leibowitch and collaborators such as J. C. Gluckman and Françoise Brun-Vézinet. Usually, lymph nodes still contain a substantial amount of virus-producing cells. However, that would not be routine for them in subsequent samples. They, too, would need to rely on the much more readily obtainable blood samples.

When we published our papers in spring 1984, four appeared in *Science*[1-4] and one in *The Lancet*.[5] We wanted to be sure we had sufficient convincing data that this was the cause of AIDS. In one of the papers, we described a total of 48 detections, or isolates, of a new retrovirus. In two other papers, we described the blood test, which was imperative for us to publish because we wanted to be sure we could have *verification*, which is necessary for scientific progress. Verification would be very difficult by virus isolation for the reasons noted above, but we were able to make the blood test simple, safe, rapid, inexpensive, and accurate: the enzyme-linked immunosorbent assay (ELISA) followed by Western blot. Verification came almost overnight on a global scale by antibodies found in the serum linked to this disease. In this period, the Montagnier group also reported virus isolates from patients with frank AIDS.

I have been asked numerous times about eureka moments. I usually respond that I had none because there was always a problem facing me the next day. One could find something up to a point and then you knew you had X, Y, and Z more to do and quickly. In other words, we had no celebrations. On the other hand, upon further reflection, I can think of two times we did find satisfaction in our progress. The first that might be described as the eureka moment was in late fall 1983. Other than finding virus in patients with AIDS and chalking up numbers to try to get convincing data that this virus was linked to AIDS, another goal was to be able to mass produce some of the isolates—that is, to grow some HIV strains in continuous culture by using immortalized (permanently growing) CD4-positive T cell lines. My technician, Betsy Read-Connole, and my coworker and friend Mika Popovic succeeded in doing this with five different strains of HIV, which we described in one of our series of papers in *Science* and *The Lancet*.[2] When this occurred, we knew something for sure: whether this virus was or was not the cause of AIDS, we were going to know within months. Why? Because we would have sufficient amounts of virus to make a global blood test (specific sera anti-HIV antibodies) possible, to obtain high-quality molecular probes, and to have the capability of detailed viral analyses. Well, so it was! This retrovirus was clearly linked to AIDS and the linkage readily verified. In fact, we might say there is more evidence that this virus causes AIDS than there is for the cause of virtually any other human disease.

A second eureka moment came after we were convinced (within our group) that we had enough data to say we had found the cause of AIDS. It is one thing, however, to be convinced within one's own research group, but to see this (prior to our publications) outside our group is another, particularly when it came from CDC.

Again, the story involves James Curran, who had sent me coded sera samples. Some were from normal, healthy donors. Others were from different AIDS patients, including samples from people with AIDS whose risk factors seemed to be a blood transfusion. We conducted the antibody test on these coded, or blinded, samples. The samples didn't just include the blood transfusion recipients of those with AIDS but also their donors, including Curran's knowledge of which of those donors subsequently developed AIDS, which is a very powerful cohort. We subsequently met for lunch on a nice, early spring day in 1984 (if memory serves) in Bethesda, Maryland, and exchanged envelopes. His included a sheet of paper that listed the diagnoses of those coded samples, which were noted with a number. My sheet of paper had the numbers with the result: positive or negative. The match was astonishing. We smiled, shook hands, and left the restaurant with good feelings. I guess you could say this was an exceptional eureka moment.

The late Jonathan Mann of the World Health Organization (WHO) described the years 1982 to 1985 as the fastest in the history of medicine, from the inception of a new and mysterious disease right up to the point where we had not only a blood test but the beginning of therapy—the latter being a historical first for a systemic viral disease with a demonstrable and objective result. That was, of course, the development of AZT by my colleague Sam Broder at the National Cancer Institute, working in collaboration with

Burroughs Wellcome. Of course, there was also detailed analysis of the genes and proteins, defined target cells, and determination of the modes of transmission. Early studies of pathogenesis also began to come from a few labs, in particular that of Tony Fauci and colleagues.

In retrospect, I think there is a critical lesson here in how we could do better, which has led me to form the Global Virus Network. The lesson is this: laboratories that moved the field the most in those early years, without exception, were working really by chance. What I mean by that is we were not "responsible." Two groups did have "responsibility": WHO and CDC. However, WHO doesn't have laboratories and doesn't know exactly what to do with a new disease of unknown origin and cannot know who to call on. CDC has an overwhelming number of responsibilities as one challenge, and the second is that although they can do great epidemiology on anything, it is hard for them to do great laboratory science on everything. And with AIDS, they didn't have anyone in the earliest stage of the epidemic who knew about retroviruses. CDC also had the advantage but also the disadvantage of being part of the US government, which often limits full global cooperation.

I believe these organizations should be complemented by a collection of *expert, responsible medical virologists* grouped together in a network throughout the world, such as the Global Virus Network, that would be able to cover every category of virus with high expertise. But that is the subject for a future story.

References

1. Gallo RC, Salahuddin SZ, Popovic M, Shearer GM, Kaplan M, Haynes BF, et al. Frequent detection and isolation of cytopathic retroviruses (HTLV-III) from patients with AIDS and at risk for AIDS. Science. 1984;224(4648):500–3.

2. Popovic M, Sarngadharan MG, Read E, Gallo RC. Detection, isolation, and continuous production of cytopathic retroviruses (HTLV-III) from patients with AIDS and pre-AIDS. Science. 1984;224(4648):497–500.

3. Sarngadharan MG, Popovic M, Bruch L, Schupbach J, Gallo RC. Antibodies reactive with human T-lymphotropic retroviruses (HTLV-III) in the serum of patients with AIDS. Science. 1984;224(4648):506–8.

4. Schupbach J, Popovic M, Gilden RV, Gonda MA, Sarngadharan MG, Gallo RC. Serological analysis of a subgroup of human T-lymphotropic retroviruses (HTLV-III) associated with AIDS. Science. 1984;224(4648):503–5.

5. Safai B, Sarngadharan MG, Groopman JE, Arnett K, Popovic M, Sliski A, et al. Seroepidemiological studies of human T-lymphotropic retrovirus type III in acquired immunodeficiency syndrome. Lancet. 1984;1(8392):1438–40.

"Slim Disease"

A New Health Scare in Uganda

DAVID SERWADDA

IN APRIL 1983, after I finished my internship in obstetrics and gynecology and in medicine at Nsambya Hospital, Kampala, I took up a position as a research fellow at the Uganda Cancer Institute (UCI) in Kampala. UCI was then the national referral center for the medical treatment of cancer. It was divided into the solid tumor wing, which mainly treated liver cancers, Kaposi's sarcoma, ovarian cancer, and breast cancer, and the lymphoma wing, which mainly managed lymphoma, namely Burkitt's lymphoma, Hodgkin's disease, and acute and chronic leukemia. I was assigned to work on the solid tumor wing.

At that time, UCI was running a journal club, where once every week we would review journal articles of interest to the Institute. Of particular interest at the time were journal articles on Kaposi's sarcoma, which was appearing in white homosexual males in California and New York who had acquired immunodeficiency syndrome, or AIDS.[1] This was of interest to us because we had a Kaposi's sarcoma treatment program. We were particularly intrigued, as Kaposi's sarcoma was not a commonly seen cancer in North America. Additionally, the clinical presentation was somewhat different from what we were seeing at UCI. The tumor lesions seen in the United States were more central—for example, on the abdomen, chest, and head. In Uganda, we would commonly see tumors in the lower limbs as a nodular or plaque form of Kaposi's sarcoma.

Interestingly, at the same time, a surgeon by the name of Ann Bayley, who was working in Lusaka Medical School in Zambia, started reporting atypical presentation of Kaposi's sarcoma among her patients. So, I also started to look for the same kind of presentation in our admitted patients at the UCI. It was remarkable that we also started to notice Kaposi's sarcoma in men and women that had a similar clinical presentation to that seen in North America. Up to this point, Kaposi's sarcoma was not commonly seen in women.

At the end of 1983, I got in touch with Ann Bayley while she was attending the East African Annual Surgeon's Conference at Kampala and had a discussion about the atypical presentation of Kaposi's sarcoma that she and I were seeing in our patients. The sociodemographics of patients at UCI differed from those of patients at Lusaka. Dr. Bayley was seeing Kaposi's sarcoma in predominantly middle-to-high socioeconomic status patients from urban areas, whereas patients at UCI were from low-income and rural backgrounds.

In early 1984, I recall reading a report in *Newsweek* magazine saying that Dr. Robert Gallo, then the head of the National Cancer Institute at the US National Institutes of Health, had isolated the cause of AIDS. This was a retrovirus referred to then as human T-lymphotropic virus III, or HTLV-III, but later named human immunodeficiency virus, or HIV. Further, Gallo reported that a rudimentary test was being developed that could demonstrate infection of HIV in an individual. This was a landmark revelation at the time. Mr. Carswell, a surgeon working at Mulago Hospital at the time, through contact with Dr. Bayley, connected us to Dr. Robert Downing, a virologist who was working in the UK. The aim was to send Dr. Downing some blood samples from our patients at UCI and see if they were infected with HIV.

Around September 1984 (three months after I sent the samples), I received an aerogramme from Dr. Downing, who was working in Salisbury, England, indicating that 4 out of about 25 blood samples I sent him from UCI were positive for HIV. Those were the first known HIV cases in Uganda.

This was a turning point in my medical career. I remember being very shocked and surprised but also somewhat excited at the same time. I was shocked because the disease that we had been reading about in magazines and journal articles was actually in our midst, but at the same time surprised, wondering how this disease could have come here so fast. And I was excited by the fact that I was about to disseminate something that would change our life for some time to come. The belief at the time was that this disease was among white male homosexuals far away in the Unites States. This was at a time when there weren't that many people moving back and forth between North America and Uganda. More striking was the fact that all the positive cases were patients coming from Rakai, a rural district in Uganda.

I remember the first person I went to talk to about this was Dr. Nelson Sewankambo, a senior lecturer at Makerere Medical School. After several discussions with Dr. Sewankambo, I was asked to present this data at the Uganda Medical Association Conference that took place in Fort Portal in late 1984. I found that people, including clinicians, were very skeptical about these cases being HIV infected, reasoning that the disease could not have arrived so quickly in Uganda. Those first four cases were published in the *British Journal of Cancer* in 1986.[2] It was one of my first publications. I was young, still a research fellow, and I had just finished my medical training. That is why I impress upon my students and young colleagues that you don't necessarily need big research funds to publish; sometimes initial observations can be of critical scientific and social value.

More Kaposi's sarcoma blood samples were sent from the UCI to the UK for HIV testing, and several turned out to be positive. In early 1984, I moved to Mulago Teaching Hospital as a senior house officer in the Department of Medicine, to start my training in internal medicine. While I was on the Internal Medicine ward, I continued to see Kaposi's sarcoma among patients who had lost a lot of weight, had recurring fevers and diarrhea, and were very sick. I kept sending blood samples to Dr. Downing from these patients on the medical wards. Once again, the striking observation from all the positive cases was that they were residents of Rakai or a neighboring district, Masaka.

On December 29, 1984, a lead article appeared on the front cover of a local daily newspaper, *The Star*, entitled "Mysterious Disease Kills 100 People in Rakai." This news article detailed a "slimming disease" that was killing people in the Rakai District. The presentation was typically fevers for months unresponsive to antimalarial medication, chronic diarrhea, and severe weight loss—thus the name "slimming." I knew immediately that this clinical presentation was the same as the HIV-positive cases I was seeing on the wards. Further, my patients lived in the Rakai or Masaka districts. I remember feeling that there was something seriously wrong going on in these districts.

Consequently, using our own money, we immediately put together an investigative team to go out to the two districts. The team included, among others, Drs. Sewankambo, Roy Mugerwa, and Ann Bailey with Robert Downing—who happened to be visiting Uganda at this point—and myself. Over two days, we examined patients in Masaka and Kalisizo Hospitals. We collected blood, sputum, urine, and stool samples to examine for viral, bacterial, parasitic, and fungal infection. We sent aliquots of the blood collected to the UK, to Dr. Downing (who had by this time returned home), for HIV testing. The results of that investigation were published in *The Lancet* in October 1985: "Slim Disease: A New Disease in Uganda and Its

Association With HTLV-III Infection."[3] That article cemented my career, as I was the first author on that article and it basically launched my career in infectious diseases.

That article generated great interest among other clinicians and epidemiologists to undertake collaborative research. Subsequently, we conducted a lot of work on the clinical manifestations of HIV. Of particular interest was the gastrointestinal[4,5] and pulmonary complication of HIV infection. Several papers were published as a result of my work in this area. We described the most common opportunistic infections observed in the gastrointestinal complication of HIV infection, noting that "slim disease," as described locally, was HIV infection with severe opportunistic infection of the gastrointestinal tract. Additionally, we observed that tuberculosis was the most common pulmonary complication of HIV infection.

The intensity and enthusiasm with which I went about undertaking my investigation and taking care of patients was very high. I was energetic, reading about everything that came in the medical literature in relation to HIV. It is worth mentioning that at that time medical journals were hard to come by in Uganda and took several months to arrive in the country. The more we investigated, the more we realized, to our astonishment, that this disease was very prevalent. We learned that there were many patients on the wards with no evidence of the classic symptoms of slim disease but who were HIV infected. Increasingly, we were getting very sick patients. Deaths on medical wards attributable to HIV infection were over 80 percent. Of particular concern were patients presenting with central nervous system symptoms. Often they had cryptococcal meningitis, and they invariably died. This was getting to be depressing and completely deflating. In Uganda, we had very little or no medication to treat opportunistic infections and often we only were able to rehydrate patients.

It slowly dawned on me that this was becoming a futile exercise. To wait for individuals to get HIV and watch them die as patients was very painful and stressful. At this point in time, we had nothing much to offer the patients. We had to do more to understand the transmission of this disease in order to prevent its acquisition.

So, in 1987 a group of us, researchers from Mulago Teaching Hospital, decided to write a proposal to enable us to study and understand more about the dynamics of HIV transmission in Rakai. We submitted our proposal to the US Centers for Disease Control for funding, which we eventually obtained from the US Agency for International Development through Columbia University. In 1988, in collaboration with Dr. Maria Wawer from Columbia University, we started a population-based cohort in the Rakai District with the primary objective of understanding the risk factors for transmission and acquisition of HIV. The main goal was pathways to the best HIV prevention strategy. This cohort later provided us with the opportunity to rigorously evaluate population-based HIV intervention and consequently reduce infection.

With this study, my career took a turn from clinical medicine to epidemiology. I became so passionately involved in population-based research that I moved from the Department of Internal Medicine to the School of Public Health in 1993. The research portfolio within this cohort has grown massively over time such that a research program, referred to as Rakai Health Sciences Program (RHSP), was established within Rakai District. Over the past 25 years, this program has contributed tremendously to our understanding of HIV transmission in rural populations in Africa. Further, it has evaluated the impact of a number of HIV interventions on HIV incidence on a population level. Recently, RHSP participated in the evaluation of the effect of male circumcision for prevention of HIV acquisition. The results of this community-based randomized trial, along with other similar studies in Africa, have had major policy implications for the control of HIV infection worldwide.

I feel a tremendous sense of satisfaction being involved in research with the ultimate aim of prevention of HIV transmission or acquisition. It turns out that this will be the most cost-effective way of controlling this epidemic.

References

1. Centers for Disease Control. Kaposi's sarcoma and *Pneumocystis* pneumonia among homosexual men—New York City and California. Morb Mortal Wkly Rep. 1981 Jul 3;30(25):305–8.

2. Serwadda D, Carswell W, Ayuko WO, Wamukoa W, Madda P, Downing RG. Further experience with Kaposi's sarcoma in Uganda. Br J Cancer. 1986;53(4):497–500.

3. Serwadda D, Mugerwa RD, Sewankambo NK, Lwegaba A, Carswell JW, Kirya GB, et al. Slim disease: a new disease in uganda and its association with HTLV-III infection. Lancet. 1985 Oct 19;2(8460):849–52.

4. Batman PA, Kapembwa MS, Miller AR, Sedgwick PM, Lucas S, Sewankambo NK, et al. HIV enteropathy: comparative morphometry of the jejunal mucosa of HIV infected patients resident in the United Kingdom and Uganda. Gut. 1998 Sep;43(3):350–5.

5. Sewankambo NK, Gray RH, Ahmad S, Serwadda D, Wabwire-Mangen F, Nalugoda F, et al. Mortality associated with HIV infection in rural Rakai District, Uganda. AIDS. 2000 Oct 20;14(15):2391–400.

Afterword

THOMAS COATES *and* WENDEE M. WECHSBERG

D URING THE FIRST DECADE OF the HIV epidemic, 65,000 people died from this disease in the United States, an ominous harbinger of what was to come. The early days of the epidemic generated much confusion about how people were infected, concern about whether or not others could be infected easily, and abundant fear, denial, and misinformation that created sensational headlines. Even though Ronald Reagan, the president between 1981 and 1989, refused to utter the word "AIDS" until 1987, many in government, academia, and communities worked hard to ensure funding for science and services.

More than three decades have passed since the beginning of the epidemic, and, incomprehensibly, an estimated 35 million people globally have died of HIV-related illnesses. Today, nearly 37 million people worldwide are living with HIV, and new incidence occurs daily.

By the end of the second decade of the epidemic, the global face of HIV was changing. The majority of people living with HIV were in sub-Saharan Africa, with over half being women of childbearing age. By the third decade, with the advent of life-saving medications, people are living longer and healthier lives, and pregnant mothers can protect their newborn babies from HIV transmission. As medications evolved, taking one pill a day for HIV became a dynamic game changer.

Collaborations between clinicians, social scientists, activists, survivors, nongovernmental entities, and governments facilitated greater understanding of the complex nature of culture, gender, and sexuality. Scientific advances also have been remarkable. In the past, clinical AIDS was a sure death sentence, with over 95 percent of people infected with HIV dying difficult deaths. Thanks to the hard work of scientists all over the world, dying from HIV no longer needs to be the case. It is remarkable that in our lifetimes, a deadly disease arrives on the scene and three decades later effective treatments are available.

This collection of narratives is a historical snapshot of when the HIV learning curve was steep. It also embodies some truly heartbreaking and uplifting personal stories that have never been told but now will not be forgotten.

Many of the contributors to this collection of narratives are still in this fight more than three decades later. As careers and lives have evolved that were committed to and passionate about eradicating this epidemic, with its multiple and intersecting complexities, many of us have become more introspective, more conscious, and wiser. Yet, along with our greater knowledge, there is an increased sense of global responsibility and concern to address the barriers surrounding HIV. For example, economic disparity—that is, poverty—brings with it many social and personal challenges and has played a devastating role in spreading HIV and in making treatment hard to access for millions of people in the United States and around the world. Also, stigma and our failure to address human sexuality challenge the urgency of prevention and treatment, especially for sexually active young people who may be unaware how HIV can ravage their lives.

Clearly, the work is not over. It was at the 11th International AIDS Conference in 1996 in Vancouver, Canada—whose theme was "One World One Hope"—that the scientists of the world announced the breakthrough findings of the effectiveness of combination therapy. But it was not until 2000, at the 13th International AIDS Conference in Durban, South Africa, that the world stood up and said that where one lives with HIV should not determine how long one lives with HIV. The theme of the 2000 conference— "Breaking the Silence"—was a big and important shout-out that the benefits of combination therapy needed to be available to everyone and especially those living in countries hardest hit by the HIV epidemic.

The Global Fund to Fight AIDS, Tuberculosis and Malaria was established in 2002, and the President's Emergency Plan for AIDS Relief (PEPFAR) was funded by President George W. Bush's administration in 2003. Since that time, scientific advances have improved treatment and given us new prevention tools. We have made progress in delivering those advances to the people who need them, with about half of the people with HIV in the world receiving treatment.

But the work is not done. The other half of the people in the world living with HIV need access to treatment. And because prevention strategies are imperfect, we need to keep working to improve treatment and prevention, including vaccines.

The stories in this book chronicle the past. We hope that they are inspiring and motivating. Now we are looking to a new cohort of committed clinicians, scientists, activists, and leaders to continue advancing science and to take those advances to every corner of the world in which they are needed. We must take our global consciousness to the next level in the ongoing fight against HIV.

There is still much critical work to do, but we are encouraged that the next generation is picking up the mantle of leadership and taking the good fight forward.

CONTRIBUTORS

QUARRAISHA ABDOOL KARIM, PhD, is an infectious diseases epidemiologist who has made seminal contributions to HIV prevention research, particularly in young women. Dr. Abdool Karim is Associate Scientific Director of CAPRISA (Centre for the AIDS Programme of Research in South Africa) and holds professorships in Clinical Epidemiology at the Mailman School of Public Health, Columbia University, and in Public Health at the Nelson R. Mandela School of Medicine, University of KwaZulu-Natal in South Africa. She is currently Vice-Chair of the South African Medical Research Council Board, a member of the UNAIDS Scientific Expert Panel, Scientific Advisor to the Executive Director of UNAIDS, an advisory board member of the Higher Education and Training HIV/AIDS Programme (HEAIDS), and Scientific Advisory Board member of PEPFAR. She is a Foreign Associate member of the US National Academy of Medicine, Fellow of the Royal Society of South Africa, Fellow of the Academy of Science of South Africa, Fellow and Vice-President (Southern African Region) of the African Academy of Sciences, and Fellow of the World Academy of Sciences.

SALIM S. ABDOOL KARIM, MBChB, PhD, DSc (honoris causa), is a clinical infectious diseases epidemiologist widely recognized for his groundbreaking scientific contributions in HIV prevention and treatment. Dr. Abdool Karim is Director of CAPRISA; Pro Vice-Chancellor (Research), University of KwaZulu-Natal; CAPRISA Professor of Global Health at Columbia University; Adjunct Professor of Medicine, Cornell University; and Associate Member of the Ragon Institute of Massachusetts General Hospital (MGH), Massachusetts Institute of Technology (MIT), and Harvard University. He currently chairs the UNAIDS Scientific Expert Panel and is a member of both the WHO HIV-TB Task Force and the WHO Expert Panel on Sexually Transmitted Infections and HIV. He is an elected Fellow of the World Academy of Sciences, African Academy of Sciences, Academy of Science in South Africa, Royal Society of South

Africa, American Academy of Microbiology, and Foreign Associate Member of the US National Academy of Medicine.

LYNDA ARNOLD, BSN, MBA, is a mother of three living children currently in the Los Angeles area. Infected with the HIV virus through an accidental needlestick in 1992 at age 23, while working in the intensive care unit at a community hospital in Lancaster, Pennsylvania, she has had a long career in healthcare, education, networking, and advocacy. Currently, she spends her time devoted to volunteering for local HIV education and case management services and as a resource parent for Los Angeles County. She enjoys supporting the activities of her young adult children in the entertainment industry and the US military. She and her husband have been married for 23 years and look forward to all of life's adventures yet to come.

ANNE JEANENE BENGOA, MS, recently earned a master's degree from the Geographic Information Science and Technology program at the University of Southern California. Additionally, she has degrees from the Universities of Miami and Maryland, in Marine Science, Biology, and Graphic Design, which alludes to the dual careers she has maintained throughout her life. She has been involved in all manner of data collection, management, analysis, display, and distribution as well as every aspect of publication, from literature reviews, writing, and editing to printing, with a focus on data visualization. Currently, Ms. Bengoa is a Research Scientist at the University of Miami, where she provides similar professional-level support for various research projects involving a wide range of issues within public health.

ROBERT E. BOOTH, PhD, is a social psychologist and Professor of Psychiatry at the University of Colorado Denver. For more than 30 years he has developed and evaluated interventions designed to prevent the spread of HIV among people who inject drugs. While the majority of this work has been in Denver, with an emphasis on assessing interventions to improve substance use treatment entry and retention, for the past 17 years he has implemented and tested behavioral interventions in Ukraine. He has more than 250 publications. Dr. Booth recently received a National Institute on Drug Abuse award to study the long-term impact of treatment entry, following three cohorts recruited between 1995 and 2012. He has served on numerous study sections for the National Institutes of Health, and from 1998 to 2002 he was a member of the Office of AIDS Research Advisory Council. He lives in unincorporated Boulder County with his wife, horses, and Labrador Retriever.

BARRY S. BROWN, PhD, spent more than 17 years with the National Institute on Drug Abuse heading up several of its branches, including the Community Research Branch, which had responsibility for administering NIDA's community-based AIDS prevention programs and studies. He currently is Adjunct Professor at the University of North Carolina–Wilmington, a Collaborating Scientist with the Institute of Behavioral Research at Texas Christian University, and a Senior Investigator with the Friends Research Institute in Baltimore, Maryland. He is the author of more than 170 articles and book chapters and coeditor of the *Handbook on Risk of AIDS*. In his spare time, he has authored four works of fiction in the *Mrs. Hudson of Baker Street* mystery series.

THOMAS COATES, PhD, is the founding director for the UCLA Center for World Health and was named the new director of the University of California Global Health Institute. Dr. Coates is the Michael and Sue Steinberg Endowed Professor of Global AIDS Research and Distinguished Professor of Medicine within the University of California, Los Angeles, Division of Infectious Diseases. His areas of emphasis and expertise are global health, HIV prevention, and its relationship to treatment and international health policy. His domestic work has focused on men who have sex with men, and he is currently finishing a nationwide clinical trial of an experimental HIV preventive intervention focused on this population. Dr. Coates is also finishing domestic trials of post-exposure prophylaxis. He has directed community-randomized clinical trials in South Africa, Zimbabwe, Tanzania, and Thailand to determine the impact of strategies for destigmatizing HIV community-wide and led a prevention clinical trial in South America as part of a five-country effort. Dr. Coates was elected to the National Academy of Medicine (formerly the Institute of Medicine) in 2000.

FRANCINE COURNOS, MD, is Professor of Clinical Psychiatry (in Epidemiology) at the Mailman School of Public Health at Columbia University and Principal Investigator of the Northeast Caribbean AIDS Education and Training Center. Dr. Cournos's career has focused on mental healthcare in the public sector, with particular attention to the interface of HIV and mental illness. This has included publishing some of the earliest studies to document elevated rates of HIV infection and associated risk behaviors among people with severe mental illness; working on numerous clinical practice guidelines and policies on HIV-related mental health issues; and participating in international efforts to integrate mental healthcare with HIV or primary care in sub-Saharan Africa, Brazil, and the Philippines. Dr. Cournos has published more than 130 articles and book chapters, the majority of which focus on mental illness and HIV.

JAMES W. CURRAN, MD, MPH, is the Dean of Public Health and an Adjunct Professor of Medicine and Nursing, and Co-Director and Principal Investigator of the Emory Center for AIDS Research. Dr. Curran is past chair of the board on Population Health and Public Health Practice of the Institute of Medicine and served on the Executive Committee of the Association of Schools of Public Health. Additionally, he holds an endowed chair at Emory University known as the James W. Curran Dean of Public Health. In 1981 Dr. Curran coordinated the task force on acquired immune deficiency syndrome (AIDS) at the Centers for Disease Control (CDC) and then led the HIV/AIDS Division. While at the CDC, he attained the rank of Assistant Surgeon General. In 1995, he was appointed professor of epidemiology and dean of the Rollins School of Public Health at Emory. Dr. Curran is a fellow of the American Epidemiologic Society, the American College of Preventive Medicine, and the Infectious Diseases Society of America.

DON C. DES JARLAIS, PhD, is Professor of Psychiatry and Preventive Medicine at the Icahn School of Medicine at Mount Sinai and Guest Investigator at Rockefeller University in New York. Dr. Des Jarlais is a leader in the fields of AIDS and injection drug use and has published extensively on these topics, including articles in the *New England Journal of Medicine*, *JAMA*, *Science*, and *Nature*. He also is active in international research. He serves as consultant to various institutions, including the Centers for Disease Control and Prevention, the National Institute on Drug Abuse, the National Academy of Sciences, and the World Health Organization. His research has received numerous awards, including a New York State Department of Health Commissioner's award for promoting the health of persons who use drugs. Formerly, Dr. Des Jarlais served as a Commissioner for the National Commission on AIDS, as a Core Group Member of the UNAIDS Reference Group on HIV and Injecting Drug Use, and as a member of the Scientific Advisory Board of the President's Emergency Plan for AIDS Relief (PEPFAR).

JEFFREY D. FISHER, PhD, is a Board of Trustees Distinguished Professor of Psychological Sciences at the University of Connecticut and the founding Director of its Institute for Collaboration on Health, Intervention, and Policy. Dr. Fisher has an extensive background in health behavior change research, health behavior change theory, and health behavior change intervention design, implementation, and evaluation and has published extensively in these domains. He is the coauthor of the Information–

Motivation–Behavioral Skills (IMB) model of health behavior change, which has been widely adopted internationally in the context of conceptual and intervention work on health behavior change. He has designed, implemented, and evaluated effective health behavior change interventions in multiple populations and health domains, with an emphasis on HIV prevention interventions in populations at risk for or living with HIV. Dr. Fisher's work has also focused on increasing medication adherence, and he has published conceptual and intervention research in this domain. His interventions have been widely disseminated.

WILLIAM A. FISHER, PhD, is Distinguished Professor, Department of Psychology and Department of Obstetrics and Gynaecology, University of Western Ontario, and Research Affiliate, Institute for Collaboration on Health, Intervention, and Policy, University of Connecticut. Dr. Fisher has been a National Health Scientist, HIV/AIDS, for Health Canada, and he is a Fellow of the Canadian Academy of Health Sciences and the Society for the Scientific Study of Sexuality. He has served as associate editor of the *Journal of Sexual Medicine* and consulting editor of *Archives of Sexual Behavior* and the *Journal of Sex Research* and received the Distinguished Scientific Contribution Award of the Society for the Scientific Study of Sexuality. Dr. Fisher has published over 200 papers concerning the social and psychological determinants of sexual and reproductive health, emphasizing theory-based research concerning prediction and promotion of HIV/AIDS preventive behavior. His work has been supported by the US National Institute of Mental Health, the Canadian Social Sciences and Humanities Research Council, and the Canadian Institute for Health Research over the past four decades.

SAMUEL R. FRIEDMAN, PhD, is Director of Infectious Disease Research at the National Development and Research Institutes, Inc., and Associate Director of the Infectious Disease, Epidemiology and Theory Core in the Center for Drug Use and HIV Research. He is an author on almost 500 publications on HIV, hepatitis C, and sexually transmitted infections, as well as drug use epidemiology and prevention. Dr. Freidman is a recipient of the NIDA Avant Garde Award (2012), the International Rolleston Award of the International Harm Reduction Association (2009), the first Sociology AIDS Network Award for Career Contributions to the Sociology of HIV/AIDS (2007), and a Lifetime Contribution Award, Association of Black Sociologists (2005). He is a long-time social justice activist as well as a multiply published poet.

ROBERT C. GALLO, MD, has been Director of the Institute of Human Virology and Professor of Medicine and Microbiology and Immunology at the

University of Maryland School of Medicine since 1996. Dr. Gallo is also currently Cofounder and Scientific Director of the Global Virus Network. Previously, he was at the National Cancer Institute. Dr. Gallo's career has focused on the study of the basic biology of human blood cells, their normal and abnormal growth, and the causes of abnormal growth and the involvement of viruses in these abnormalities. He and his coworkers opened and pioneered the field of human retrovirology in 1980 when they discovered the first human retrovirus, HTLV-1, and with others, showed it was a cause of a particular form of human leukemia. A year later, he and his group discovered the second known human retrovirus, HTLV-2. Dr. Gallo and colleagues developed the lifesaving HIV blood test in 1983–1984.

MARY GUINAN, MD, PhD, is a physician and scientist who worked for the Centers for Disease Control for 24 years as a medical epidemiologist and administrator. Dr. Guinan served in the worldwide smallpox eradication program in India and was part of the CDC team that investigated the early AIDS epidemic. She was the first woman to serve as the CDC's Associate Director for Science, the chief scientific advisor to the Director of CDC. Her work in AIDS is documented in the book and movie *And the Band Played On* by Randy Shilts. In 1998, she left CDC and was appointed the Nevada State Health Officer. In 2004, she became the founding Dean of the School of Public Health (since renamed the School of Community Health Sciences) at the University of Nevada, Las Vegas (UNLV). She retired from UNLV in 2014. In 2014, she was awarded the Elizabeth Blackwell Medal from the American Medical Women's Association for outstanding contributions to medicine and science. Her first book, *Adventures of a Female Medical Detective*, was published by Johns Hopkins University Press in 2016.

GIBBIE HARRIS, MSPH, BSN, is a founding partner/consultant of Praxis Partners for Health and most recently was the Health Director for Buncombe County, North Carolina. Ms. Harris retired from county government after 25 years in local public health, most of that time as a local health director. Currently, her consultation work includes working with hospital systems, local and state health departments, free clinics, and communities. Her experience and expertise provide support in the areas of systems and community development, strategic planning, organizational and leadership capacity building, and local health department leadership and management. She currently serves on the National Association of City and County Health Officers' Public Health Transformation and Public Health Communication Committees, the NC Family Nurse Practitioner Advisory Council, the YMCA of Western North Carolina Board, and the Verner Early Childhood Development Board.

WARREN W. HEWITT JR., DrPH, MS, is presently the CEO of HKJ Behavioral Health Services, LLC, in Baltimore, Maryland. Before retirement in 2014, Dr. Hewitt was the Senior Health Advisor on HIV to the Director of the Center for Substance Abuse Treatment in the US Department of Health and Human Services. From 2003 to 2004, he was Senior Health Policy Advisor to the Director of the Office of Demand Reduction in the White House Office of National Drug Control. He also served as the Associate Director of the Office of Minority Health from 1986 to 1989 and as a Health Policy Analysis Officer in the Office of the Assistant Secretary for Planning and Evaluation. Aside from government appointments, Dr. Hewitt also has held various research positions at George Washington University, the California Institute of Technology, the Jet Propulsion Laboratory, and Springfield College.

SUSAN M. KEGELES, PhD, is Professor of Medicine at the University of California, San Francisco, School of Medicine, in the Division of Prevention Science and Co-Director of the Center for Prevention Studies. Dr. Kegeles has an established research career conducting community-based research and has considerable experience designing and implementing HIV prevention interventions for diverse groups, including young and all-aged men who have sex with men, transgender women, and injection drug users. She developed the Mpowerment Project, an efficacious multilevel HIV prevention intervention that works at the level of the community and addresses individual, interpersonal, social, and structural issues related to HIV prevention. The Mpowerment Project has been implemented by over 300 community-based organizations in the US, as well as internationally in South Africa, Peru, Mexico, Guatemala, Canada, the Netherlands, Hong Kong, and Beirut. Dr. Kegeles is currently conducting research on mobilizing young MSM communities to influence engagement in the HIV continuum of care and prevention in the US South, South Africa, and Peru.

RAYFORD KYTLE began his work in 1986, focused on AIDS at the US Department of Health and Human Services. From 2005 to 2013, he was a writer/editor for the Division of AIDS Research at the National Institute of Mental Health. As a gay man, he lived in New York City from 1975 to 1980. He tested positive for HIV as soon as the test was made available in September 1984. He was the primary caregiver for his two partners, who died due to complications resulting from AIDS. Despite a deteriorating immune system, which in 1993 reached the level of full-blown AIDS, and numerous serious side effects, he has never been disabled. Since retiring in 2013, he has focused on writing about his life as a gay man, in hopes that it may benefit others growing up in similar circumstances. Lately, he has also been focused on activism.

BISHOP STACEY S. LATIMER is a native of Laurens, South Carolina, where his ministry began. He is currently Founder/Spiritual Leader of Love Alive International Sanctuary of Praise Worship Center of New York City (LAISP) and Founder/CEO of Love Alive International Foundation (LAIF), headquartered in New York City. He is a proud veteran of the United States Army. Bishop Latimer is the Faith-based Director for the New York City Faith in Action Coalition for HIV/AIDS (NYCFIA). He is the Faith Coordinator and Chaplain for Watchful Eye. He is a member of the African American Clergy and Elected Officials Coalition. Bishop Latimer works closely with the New York City Department of Health and Mental Hygiene's Center for Health Equity and HIV/AIDS Faith Initiatives, both city and statewide. He is a 30-plus year survivor of an HIV diagnosis. His work and ministry has impact across the globe. He understands the need to prioritize AIDS in every community until there's a cure.

ROBERT LOVE is a native Californian, born and raised in Southern California. He moved to the city of San Francisco in 1970, and the City has been his home ever since. He owns a landscape design firm in Sausalito and is also Managing Director of a small community theater in the North Bay. He resides in the Sunset District of San Francisco with his husband.

DUANE C. MCBRIDE, PhD, is Professor of Sociology at Andrews University and Director of the University's Institute for Prevention of Addictions. He holds a doctorate in sociology from the University of Kentucky. Dr. McBride has published over 100 articles, chapters, and monographs in health services research, the etiology and health consequences of substance abuse, and program evaluation. He was involved in early research on the risk factors associated with HIV infection among injecting drug users that was published in the *American Journal of Public Health* and other venues. His research has been supported by the National Institute on Drug Abuse, the Robert Wood Johnson Foundation, and the National Institute of Justice. He currently serves as a grant reviewer for the National Institutes of Health and a consultant to the University of Michigan's Monitoring the Future Project. His current research interests include service program evaluation and drug policy analysis.

CLYDE B. MCCOY, PhD, has assisted the University of Miami in many and varied capacities over the past 40 years, including serving as the Director of the Comprehensive Drug Research Center (CDRC) and the Health Services Research Center (HSRC). These centers have produced 12 academic chairs serving varied public health fields. Dr. McCoy was also Chair of the Department of Epidemiology and Public Health from 1997 to 2009. During his academic research career he focused on both national and international research in multiple disciplines in the public health field—specifically, community studies, sociology, demography, epidemiology, addiction sciences, and health services research. His research includes substantive publications on migrants and on various epidemiological areas, including cancer, drug abuse, HIV, hepatitis, and AIDS. He has brought a unique approach to research and mentoring over four decades of international collaboration and research.

CARMEN MORRIS currently works in a local grocery store in her small hometown. She's also taking some online classes at a community college down the road from where she lives because she still hasn't decided what she wants to do when she grows up. In some time, she hopes that her writing will be enough to start some kind of career, but she doesn't know what the future will bring. As for now, she currently has the cutest dog, she lives happily with her childhood best friend, and she takes in all the short-lived moments around her as she waits for the future to arrive.

WILLO PEQUEGNAT, PhD, spent 26 years in the AIDS Program at the National Institute of Mental Health (NIMH), National Institutes of Health. Because of the generous congressional funding for this emerging but poorly understood epidemic, she was able to shape an important national and international behavioral AIDS research program by writing announcements to elicit research proposals. She served as a staff investigator on four cutting-edge clinical trials. Since reluctantly leaving NIMH, she has formed her own company, Salix Health Consulting, Inc., and engages specifically in projects that are of current interest to her, such as developing a model of an evidence-based prevention program to prevent or reduce mortality and morbidity in mothers and children in the developing world, and developing an interactive online 15-session workshop to provide technical assistance to ethnic minority investigators.

MARY JANE ROTHERAM-BORUS, PhD, has spent the past 30 years developing, evaluating, and disseminating evidence-based interventions for children and families. She has worked extensively with adolescents, especially those at risk for substance use, HIV, homelessness, depression, suicide, and long-term unemployment. She has directed and implemented several landmark intervention studies that have demonstrated the benefits of providing behavior change programs and support to families in risky situations. Several of these programs have received national and international recognition, including designation as model programs by the American Psychological Association, the American Medical Association, the Centers for Disease Control and Prevention, and the Substance Abuse and Mental Health Services Administration. Dr. Rotheram-Borus has initiated projects in Thailand, India, Uganda, China, South Africa, and the United States. She has authored or coauthored more than 375 journal articles, including publications in *Science*, *JAMA*, and the *American Journal of Public Health*. In 2000, 2001, and 2007, *Science* identified Dr. Rotheram-Borus among the top NIH-funded researchers for investigator-initiated grants.

JEFFREY SAMET, MD, is the John Noble Professor of Medicine and Professor of Public Health at Boston University School of Medicine and a practicing primary care physician at Boston Medical Center, with expertise treating substance use disorders in general healthcare settings and researching the impact of substance use on HIV infection. Dr. Samet is Chief of General Internal Medicine at Boston University School of Medicine/Boston Medical Center and Vice Chair for Public Health in the Department of Medicine. He is Editor of the journal *Addiction Science & Clinical Practice*. He is Principal Investigator of the National Institute on Alcohol Abuse and Alcoholism (NIAAA) Alcohol-HIV Consortium, URBAN ARCH, and two National Institute on Drug Abuse R25 grants to advance physician addiction education and research: the Chief Residents Immersion Training (CRIT) Program and the Research in Addiction Medicine Scholars (RAMS) Program, which advance research careers for addiction subspecialty physicians. Dr. Samet's international HIV work has occurred predominantly in Russia but also in India, Uganda, Ukraine, and Vietnam.

DAVID SERWADDA, MBChB, MMed, MPH, has more than 23 years' experience working in the field of evaluating population-based HIV interventions, and care and treatment of AIDS. Dr. Serwadda is professor of infectious disease in the department of Disease Control and Environmental Health, Makerere University School of Public Health, Uganda, and a former Dean of the School, as well as Executive Director of Rakai Health Science Program (RHSP) for the past 20 years. In this role, he has been involved in the design, implementation, and analysis of population-based HIV intervention in a rural district in Rakai, Uganda. He is a founding member of the Makerere University School of Public Health Fellowship Program. Professor Serwadda received his medical degree, MBChB, and Master of Internal Medicine, MMed, from Makerere University and an MPH and honorary doctorate from Johns Hopkins Bloomberg School of Public Health. He has been inducted as a member of the Johns Hopkins University Society of Scholars and is also a member of the Institute of Medicine.

LORRAINE SHERR, PhD, is based at University College London. Professor Sherr is the editor of several international journals, including *AIDSCare*, *Psychology, Health & Medicine*, and *Vulnerable Children and Youth Studies*. She has authored over 270 academic papers and more than 40 texts. She sits on the International Committee of AIDSImpact and several IAS International Conferences. She is an invited adjunct professor at the Chinese University of Hong Kong and has served on various international initiatives, such as the Joint International Learning Initiative on Children and AIDS (JLICA), the WHO Disclosure group, and the WHO Strategic Advisory Council (STAC) on AIDS. Prof. Sherr has worked with NORAD/SIDA–Norway Sweden, the World Bank, Harvard University, REPSSI: Regional Psychosocial Support Programme, Amsterdam Cohort Study International Organizations (such as World Vision, Save the Children, Care International, HelpAge, and the Bernard Van Leer Foundation), and Harvard University in partnership with global groups such as JLICA and Know Violence. She has a broad portfolio of national and international research focused mostly on families and HIV.

JAMES L. SORENSEN, PhD, has made significant contributions to the treatment of HIV among people with addiction and co-occurring disorders over the past 30 years. Dr. Sorensen serves as professor in residence in the University of California, San Francisco, Department of Psychiatry at Langley Porter Psychiatric Institute and as part of the medical staff at Zuckerberg San Francisco General Hospital, in which he dedicates much of his research to treatment and services in substance abuse and community mental health. He serves as Co-director of the Western States Node of the National Drug Abuse Treatment Clinical Trials Network. In addition to his own research, he continues to mentor many budding researchers who have an interest in working in these fields.

JACK B. STEIN, PhD, is the Director of the Office of Science Policy and Communications at the National Institute on Drug Abuse (NIDA), part of the National Institutes of Health. Dr. Stein possesses over two decades of professional experience in leading national drug and HIV-related research, practice, and policy. He has held other positions at NIDA, including Deputy Director for the Division of Epidemiology, Services and Prevention Research. Prior to NIDA, he served as the Chief of the Prevention Branch, Office of Demand Reduction, at the White House Office of

National Drug Control Policy and as Director, Division of Services Improvement within the Substance Abuse and Mental Health Services Administration.

CHARLES VAN DER HORST, MD, FACP, is Emeritus Professor of Medicine and Infectious Diseases at the University of North Carolina at Chapel Hill. His career encompassed clinical medicine, National Institutes of Health–funded clinical research, teaching, and implementing clinical and research programs. From 1986 to 2000, his focus was the AIDS epidemic in the United States, and from 2001 to 2017, the AIDS epidemic in Africa. He currently serves as a volunteer primary care physician at a free clinic in North Carolina and technical advisor for More Than Me, a nongovernmental organization in Liberia. He also serves as a senior advisor to the UNC Fogarty Global Health Fellows Consortium. Dr. van der Horst has been an activist for many years, including being arrested for civil disobedience in 2013 at the North Carolina legislature, protesting their refusal to expand Medicaid, helping to halt executions in North Carolina in 2006, organizing, and writing political editorials.

WENDEE M. WECHSBERG, PhD, is Director and Principal Researcher for the Substance Use, Gender, and Applied Research Program at RTI International. Dr. Wechsberg is also the Founding Director of the RTI Global Gender Center. She is Adjunct Professor at the University of North Carolina at Chapel Hill Gillings School of Global Public Health, Adjunct Professor of Psychology at North Carolina State University, and Adjunct Professor in Psychiatry and Behavioral Medicine at Duke University School of Medicine. Dr. Wechsberg started her career in 1977 as an addiction clinician and treatment director. She is the creator of the woman-focused HIV prevention program the Women's CoOp, a Centers for Disease Control and Prevention best-evidence HIV behavioral prevention intervention. The Women's CoOp has been adapted specifically for underserved and vulnerable adult and adolescent women in the United States and in international settings. Dr. Wechsberg has been a National Institutes of Health principal investigator focused on gender, substance use, and HIV prevention since 1994. She was ranked third among all NIH-funded AIDS researchers in 2008.

WAYNE WIEBEL, PhD, is Professor Emeritus in Epidemiology at the University of Illinois at Chicago School of Public Health. Upon joining the faculty in 1986, he founded the school's Community Outreach Intervention Program to conduct research on and mobilize intervention services targeting the emergent HIV/AIDS epidemic among injection drug users. This laid the foundation for what would later be published in over 10 languages as *The Indigenous Leader Outreach Intervention Manual* and adapted in numerous settings around the world as a framework for launching HIV/AIDS intervention programming.

WILLIAM A. ZULE, DrPH, began his research career in 1989 at the University of Texas Health Science Center at San Antonio, shortly after completing his bachelor's degree. Dr. Zule started as the ethnographer for the San Antonio site of the National AIDS Demonstration Research (NADR) Program, which was the first major HIV prevention initiative funded by the National Institute on Drug Abuse. He completed his DrPH in 1996 while working as the Project Director for the San Antonio site of NIDA's Cooperative Agreement for AIDS Community-Based Outreach/ Intervention Research Program. Dr. Zule's early work helped call attention to the social context of indirect sharing practices and differences between people who injected heroin and methamphetamine. He also examined the effects of different syringe designs on HIV transmission. He currently serves as a board member and is the former President of the North Carolina Harm Reduction Coalition. Dr. Zule is currently a Senior Research Health Analyst in the Substance Use, Gender, and Applied Research Program at RTI International and an RTI Fellow.

Note: Page numbers followed by *f* indicate figures.

LAV (lymphadenopathy-associated virus), 39
Lazarus, Jeff, 135
Lazarus effect, 202
Lebanon, 135, 137
Leibowitch, Jacques, 218
leukoencephalopathy, progressive multifocal, 112
Levine, Ron, 70
Lewin, Kurt, 191
Lewis, C. S., 3
Lira, Armando, 156–160
listening to the patient, 12–13
Los Angeles, California, 55, 148
Lusaka Medical School, 221
lymphadenopathy, 39

Madden, Annie, 164
Maddux, Fred, 141
Malaria Surveillance Program, KwaZulu-Natal, 78
Mandela, Nelson, 80
Mann, Jonathan, xiv, 219–220
marginalization, 60
Marmor, Mike, 179
Maryland Department of Health and Mental Hygiene, 128
Masaka Hospital, 223
Maslansky, Robert, 179
Mata, Alberto, 174
Mbeki, Thabo, 80
McKinnon, Karen, 24
McKusick, Leon, 134
MDHG, Amsterdam, the Netherlands, 163–164
Medical Research Council (MRC), South Africa, 78, 81
Medicare, 51
medication assistance programs, 32
medications: adherence to, 51–54, 74–75; regimens, 203; side effects of, 46–47, 50–52, 54
Memory and Aging Center, University of California, San Francisco, 54
Memory Boxes, 61
mentally ill patients, 22–27
methadone treatment, 70–76, 147–149
Mfume, Kweisi, 102
Miami, Florida, 206–207, 211

Miami-Dade County, Florida, 207–211, 207f–210f
microbicides, 78–79, 82–83
Microbicide Trials Network, 82
Middle East, drug users' groups, 165
Mildvan, Donna, 38–39, 179
Millett, Greg, 136
Minority HIV/AIDS Initiative, 9–10
Moattie, Jean Paul, 69
mobilization, 98–99
Moe, Ardis, 53, 56
Montagnier, Luc, 35–36, 38, 40, 181, 217–218
Montlanthe, Kgalema, 80
Moodley, Jack, 81
Moore, Douglas, 116
Morbidity and Mortality Weekly Report (*MMWR*), 37, 133, 178
Mosby, Roosevelt, 136
Moss, Andrew, 148–149
mothers with AIDS, 59–60
Motsoaledi, Aron, 81
Mount Zion Baptist Missionary Baptist Church, Laurens, SC, 96
Mpowerment Project, 135–137
Mugerwa, Roy, 223
Mulago Hospital, 222
Mulago Teaching Hospital, 223–225
multifocal leukoencephalopathy, progressive, 112
Murphy, Eddie, 111

NAACP (National Association for the Advancement of Colored People), US, 102
National AIDS Behavioral Survey, US, 201
National AIDS Demonstration Research (NADR) project, US, 138–139, 152, 154, 160, 172–177
National Association of People with AIDS, US, 111, 193
National Black Leadership Commission on AIDS, US, 99–100, 103
National Cancer Institute, US, 36, 219–220
National Caucus of Black State Legislators, US, 103

National Commission on AIDS, US, 176, 183
National Conclave on HIV/AIDS Policy for Black Clergy, US, 103
National Conference of Black Mayors, US, 103
National Health Service, UK, 66
National HIV/AIDS and Sexually Transmitted Infection Programme, South Africa, 79
National Holistic Institute, US, 118
National Institute of Allergy and Infectious Diseases, US, 200
National Institute of Communicable Diseases, US, 81
National Institute of Mental Health (NIMH), US, 24, 58, 134, 190–192, 197, 199–204
National Institute on Alcohol Abuse and Alcoholism, US, 73
National Institute on Drug Abuse (NIDA), US, 72–73, 129–130, 152–153, 165, 174–178, 206, 208–209; Community Epidemiology Work Group (CEWG), 150, 153; Cooperative Agreement for HIV AIDS risk-reduction studies, xv; HIV/AIDS programming, 138, 171–172; needle exchange grants, 173–174; *Research in Progress,* 141
National Institutes of Health (NIH), US, 35–36, 79, 109, 113, 167, 200, 202–203; AIDS grants, 72, 206; Comprehensive International Program of Research on AIDS, 81
National Medical Association, US, 103
National Minority AIDS Council (NMAC), US, 7
Needle, Richard, 174–175
needle exchange programs, 75, 165, 173–174, 183
needles: detachable, 142; protected, 47
needle sharing, 66, 141, 181, 183. *See also* syringe-mediated drug sharing
needlestick accidents, 44–48, 50–51
Nemeth-Coslett, Ro, 174–175
Nesbit, Sammy, 136
Netherlands, 162–168
Neupogen, 54

neurocognitive disorder, mild, 48–49
New England Journal of Medicine, 62
New Federalism, 6
Newman, Robert, 180
Newsweek, 222
New York City, 98–99, 148, 173, 179, 181, 183; Commission on AIDS, 183; Department of AIDS Services, 59–60
New York State Commission on AIDS, 183
New York State Office of Drug Abuse Services, 178–179, 182–183
New York State Office of Mental Health (NYSOMH), 22–27
New York State Psychiatric Institute, 23–24
New York Times, 108, 173–174, 186
Nixon, Richard M., 172, 200
Nobel Prize in Medicine, 35–36, 41
non-nucleoside reverse transcriptase inhibitor (NNRTI) drugs, 9
nonoxynol-9, 78–79
North Africa, drug users' groups, 165
North American Syringe Exchange Network, 164
North Carolina, 29, 70–73, 75
North Central Bronx Hospital, 17
Novick, David, 182
Nsambya Hospital, 221
nurses, 44–56
Nyswander, Marie, 179

Obama, Barack, 130
Ockham's razor, 18
Office of AIDS Research, 60
Office of National Drug Control Policy, 130
Office of the Assistant Secretary for Health (OASH), Department of Health and Human Services, 113
Oliver, Kathy, 183
Ouellet, Lawrence, 160

Pacific drug users' groups, 165
pain management, 54
Palsgrove, Gary, 174–175
parenteral nutrition, 53–54
parsimony, 18
patient-doctor relationships, 12–16

University of California, San Francisco (UCSF), 54, 58, 133–134
University of California Medical Center (UCMC), 116–117
University of Cape Town, 81
University of Illinois at Chicago, 129
University of Miami, 205–206, 211
University of Natal, 77–78, 81
University of North Carolina (UNC), 31
University of North Carolina at Chapel Hill, 73
University of Texas, San Antonio (UTSA), 139–140
University of Texas School of Public Health (UTSPH), 140
University of Western Cape, 81
US Agency for International Development (USAID), 224–225
users' groups, 162–168, 183
US Public Health Service (USPHS), 7, 113

vaginal microbicides, 78, 82–83
Vancouver Area Network of Drug Users, 165
van den Boom, Frans, 69
Vezinet-Brun, Francoise, 41–42
Vietnam, 41
Vincent, Will, 136
VOICE (Vaginal and Oral Interventions to Control the Epidemic) trial, 82
voluntary counseling and testing (VCT), 202
Votsberger, Ken, 139
Vulcan Gas Company, 138

Wake County, North Carolina, 28–30
Wake Health Services, 31
Wake Medical Center, 29, 31
Walter Reed Army Medical Center, 93, 95

Walters, Heather, 58
Ward, Doug, 113
Washington Heights Community Service, 23
Waters, Maxine, 9–10, 92
Watters, John, 150–151
Wawer, Maria, 224–225
Waxman, Henry, 176
Webber, Randall, 153
Weissman, Gloria, 174
Wellcome Trust, 81
Wheeler, Daryl, 136
White, Ryan, 98
Whitman Walker Clinic, 112
Wiebel, Wayne, 150–151, 175–176
Wikipedia, 36
Williams, Robert, 136
Windsor, Isobel, 77
Wolvaardt, Gustaaf, 79
woman-focused interventions, 73
women: African American, 72–73, 193; HIV prevention in young, 77–85; mothers with AIDS, 59–60; who use drugs, 70–76
Women's (Health) CoOp, 73–74
workers' compensation, 46–51, 55
World Health Organization (WHO), xiv, 82, 142, 164, 183, 219–220

Yancovitz, Stan, 179
YMCA, 107, 110
young women, HIV prevention in, 77–85
youth with HIV, 121–124
YouTube, 38

Zambia, 221
zidovudine (AZT), 14, 59, 77, 93, 201, 219–220
Zika virus, 63
Zuma, Jacob, 80

Library of Congress Cataloging-in-Publication Data

Names: Wechsberg, Wendee M., editor.
Title: HIV pioneers : lives lost, careers changed, and survival / edited by Wendee M.
   Wechsberg; foreword by James W. Curran.
Description: Baltimore : Johns Hopkins University Press, 2018. | Includes
   bibliographical references and index.
Identifiers: LCCN 2017046661| ISBN 9781421425726 (pbk. : alk. paper) |
   ISBN 1421425726 (pbk. : alk. paper) | ISBN 9781421425733 (electronic) |
   ISBN 1421425734 (electronic)
Subjects: | MESH: HIV Infections—history | Acquired Immunodeficiency Syndrome—
   history | Biomedical Research—history | HIV Long-Term Survivors | History,
   20th Century | Personal Narratives
Classification: LCC RC607.A26 | NLM WC 503 | DDC 616.97/92—dc23
LC record available at https://lccn.loc.gov/2017046661